Holistic Healing

HOLISTIC HEALING

An Hachette UK Company
www.hachette.co.uk

Vie Books, an imprint of Summersdale Publishers Ltd
Part of Octopus Publishing Group Limited
Carmelite House
50 Victoria Embankment
LONDON
EC4Y 0DZ
UK

www.summersdale.com

Printed and bound in China

ISBN: 978-1-78783-648-8

Substantial discounts on bulk quantities of Summersdale books are available to corporations, professional associations and other organizations. For details contact general enquiries: telephone: +44 (0) 1243 771107 or email: enquiries@summersdale.com.

Neither the author nor the publisher can be held responsible for any loss or claim arising out of the use, or misuse, of the suggestions made herein. It's always advisable to consult a physician before beginning a new exercise regime or diet.

Sally Brockway

Holistic Healing

Live Your Best Life the Natural Way

vie

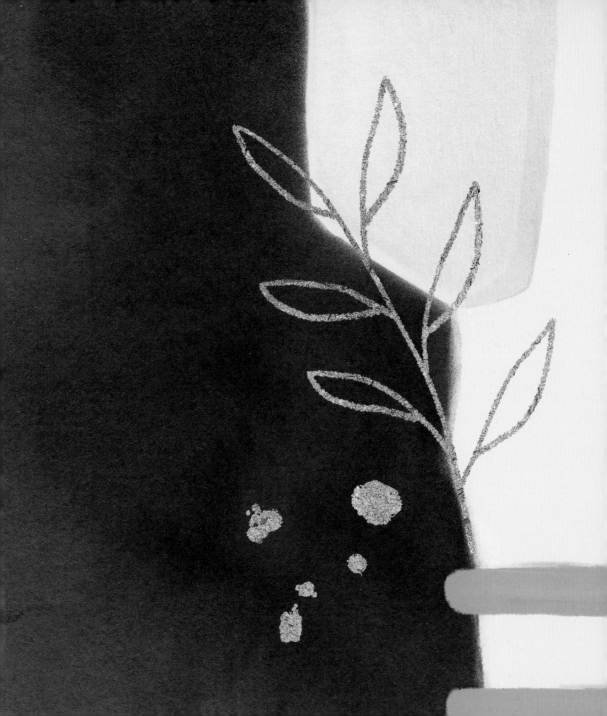

Contents

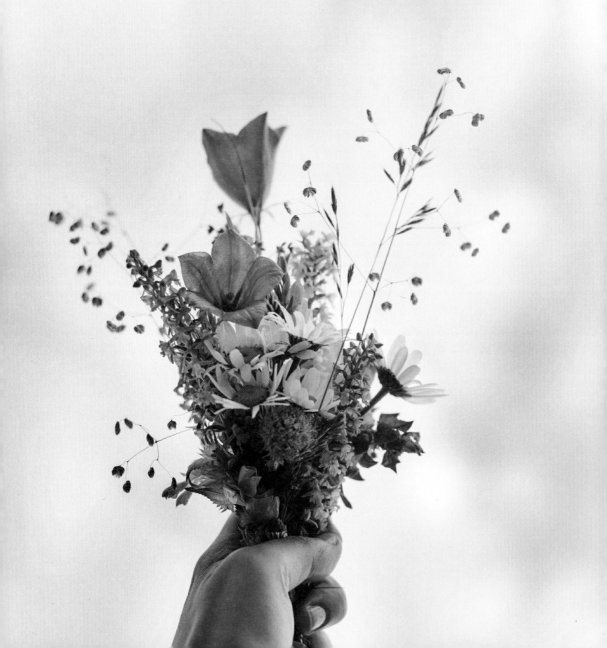

Introduction

Holistic healing is a form of medicine that takes every aspect of a person into consideration rather than focusing on the specific symptoms of an illness. It comes from the word "holism'" which means "relating to the whole" and is the foundation upon which all ancient healing traditions are built.

According to holistic healing principles, in order to function as your very best self, the mind, body and soul need to be in perfect harmony. What goes on in the outside world matters too, as our environment, where we live, our workplace and the people we interact with are all part of the equation. If just one aspect is out of kilter, all of you suffers.

Treating any illness with holistic methods involves finding the root cause of the condition, whether it is emotional, physical, spiritual or environmental, and while there are many brilliant holistic healers operating all over the world, the practice relies on each of us taking responsibility for our own wellness. The belief that we can heal ourselves is at the core of holistic healing.

This means we must practise self-love and ensure that our health and well-being is a priority. It requires that we slow down and pay attention to what is going on in our heart, mind and body. We also need to eat well, exercise regularly and get enough sleep on a daily basis.

It is believed that holistic healing began before records were introduced and cave paintings show that plants were used as medicine as far back as 25,000 BC. The practice has remained popular thanks to the centuries' worth of evidence that prove it works.

Throughout the pages of this book, you will be given an overview of all aspects of holistic healing, some of which may already be familiar to you. It is recommended that you read from start to finish and try anything that resonates along the way.

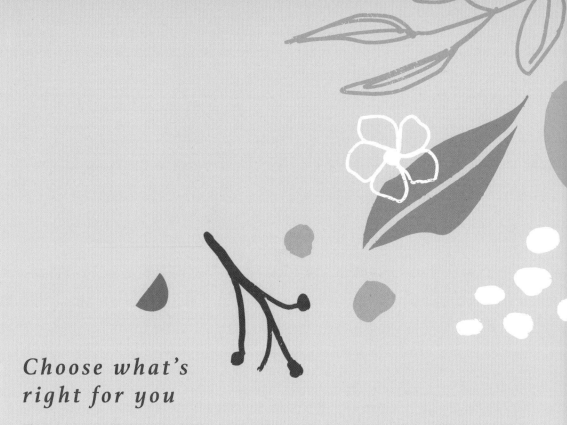

Choose what's right for you

There are many things you can do at home to enhance your health and well-being, and the trick is to find the approach – or combination of approaches – that is right for you. As you try out the various ideas in this book, you'll know which ones are a match made in heaven when you feel energized and more joyful while doing them. Don't be afraid to try new things, because sometimes we don't know what really lights us up until we have a go.

With any new pursuit, it is worth trying it for at least seven days before writing it off. If it's still not helping, see if you can adapt it to suit your tastes, or move on and try something else.

If you already have a passion or hobby, then you can use it for holistic purposes. For example, if you like painting, try to do it mindfully and don't worry about the final outcome. The same goes for cooking, sewing, crafting and even exercise. Commit to giving all of you to every activity and fully immerse yourself in the moment, because at the end of the day it's all you have.

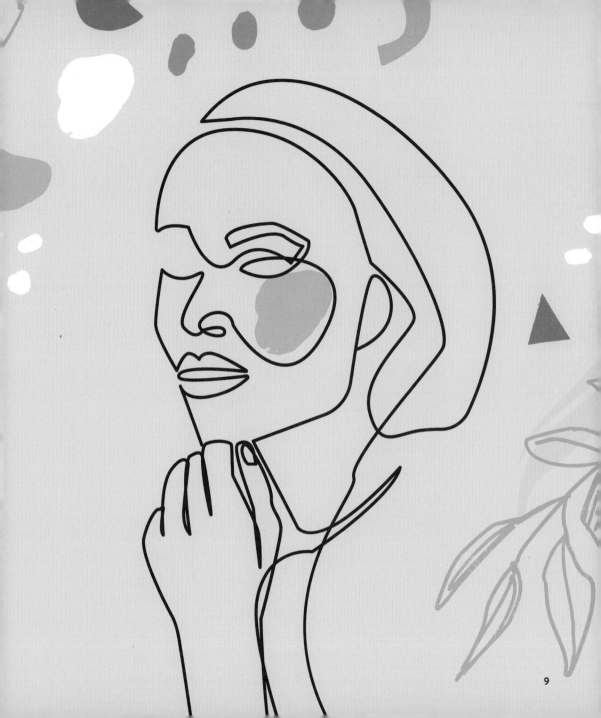

I have the
power to stay
well in mind,
body and soul

It is more important to know what sort of person has a disease than to know what sort of disease a person has.

Hippocrates

Chapter One

Traditional Holistic Practices

Most traditional holistic practices are based on knowledge and experience that has been passed down over thousands of years. There are many different types of holistic therapies and the best approach is to find the one that suits you. They all follow the basic principle of considering any illness as something that is caused by an upset in the mind, body and soul balance. The holistic healer sees themselves as one who restores harmony as opposed to targeting specific symptoms, and treatments are generally gentle and safe.

The doctor of the future will give no medicine, but will interest his patients in the care of the human frame, in diet and in the cause and prevention of disease.

Thomas Edison

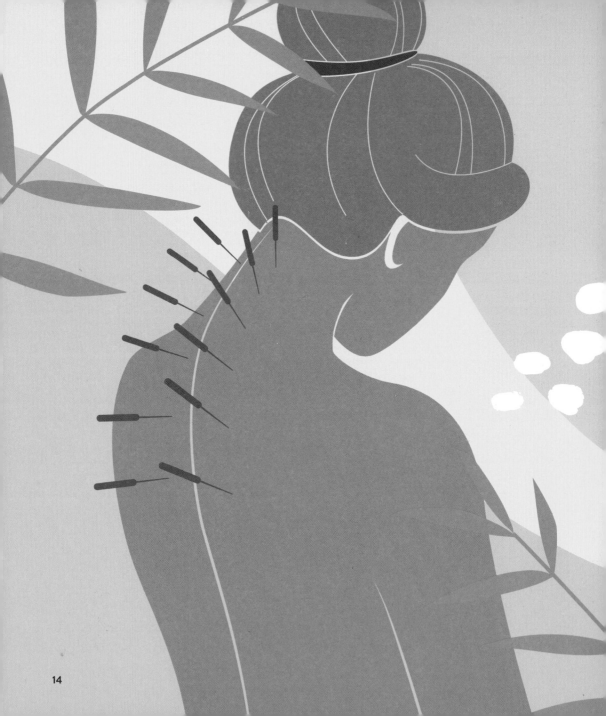

Acupuncture

Acupuncture has been practised in China for more than 2,500 years and is based on the premise that there are energy patterns flowing through the body that must be balanced if we are to achieve optimum wellness. This energy is known as qi (pronounced "chee").

Qi flows through the body along invisible channels called meridians and each of these corresponds to different organs and parts of the body. Along them lie acupoints where the qi is closer to the surface of the skin where it can be more easily manipulated.

An acupuncture session lasts for between 60–90 minutes. After an assessment and examination, you'll be asked to remove some clothing and lie down. Then, sterilized fine needles are placed under the skin into the acupoints that correspond to the issues requiring treatment.

Each of the needles causes a minute injury to the body, which is just enough to let it know that a response is called for. The body reacts by stimulating immune, healing and pain relief systems. It is not painful and when done by a qualified acupuncture practitioner, it is perfectly safe. Research has shown that acupuncture is particularly effective in the treatment of lower back pain and headaches, and can also aid sleep and ease joint pain. Everyone reacts differently to acupuncture, but most people report that they feel energized, relaxed and more balanced after a session.

Acupressure

Like acupuncture, acupressure works on the belief that energy, aka qi, flows through our bodies. Rather than insert needles to stimulate acupoints, practitioners apply pressure with the fingers, rollers or a small rubber ball. When pressure is applied to the acupoints, it unclogs the energy, releases muscular tension and stimulates blood flow.

It can be an effective form of pain relief as natural painkilling chemicals in our bodies are released when acupressure points are stimulated. It is also beneficial as a stress reliever, and can help with weight loss and to heal emotional issues.

There are different types of acupressure massage including:

- Tui na – a form of Chinese massage where acupressure points are stimulated using knuckles, palms, fingers and thumbs.

- Shiatsu – an ancient Japanese massage technique where the hands, legs, arms and feet are used to apply pressure.

- Su jok – South Korean therapy, which focuses on acupoints in the hands and feet.

Prior to a session, an acupressure therapist will do an assessment to find out which type is right for you and which acupoints need the most focus. The treatment is done fully clothed and lasts between 30–60 minutes.

You can also use acupressure yourself at home. Here are some of the points you can work on with your fingers and thumbs:

- Hollow of your inner ankle – massage to relieve menstrual cramps.

- Spot between the eyebrows – rub in circles to help with insomnia.

- Space between the nose and upper lip – press to relieve lower back pain.

- Muscle between thumb and index finger – apply pressure to relieve headaches.

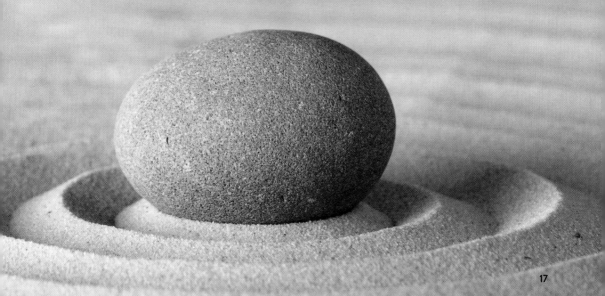

Ayurveda

Ayurveda originated in India and the word means "science of life". It is one of the world's oldest holistic practices, placing emphasis on the prevention of illness rather than symptom relief.

The two basic principles of Ayurveda, according to Deepak Chopra, author, doctor and pioneer of integrated medicine, are that the mind and body are inextricably linked, and that nothing has more power to heal and transform the body than the mind.

The Ayurvedic tradition calls for: meditation to calm the mind; for the diet to be nutritious and the digestive system aided by sitting for meals, eating slowly, minimizing raw foods and drinking hot water with lemon and ginger; and practising some form of gentle exercise.

In Ayurvedic medicine, each person is seen as having three types of energy that work together:

1. **Vata** – breathing, heart and all movements in the cells. Promotes – creativity and flexibility. Imbalance – produces fear and anxiety.

2. **Pitta** – the digestive system. Promotes – understanding and intelligence. Imbalance – can lead to anger, hatred and jealousy.

3. **Kapha** – bones, muscles and tendons. Promotes – love and forgiveness. Imbalance – can lead to greed and envy.

People are divided into types, depending on their dominant energy force. These types are called **doshas** and there are three of them. Most people are a mix of all three energies and it is the dominant type that defines your dosha.

1. **Vata** types should keep warm, stay calm, avoid cold or raw foods, eat warm foods and spices, develop a routine and get enough rest.

2. **Pitta** types should avoid excessive heat, oil and steam, limit salt intake and eat cooling foods.

3. **Kapha** types should exercise well, avoid heavy foods, stay active, avoid dairy, oil and fatty foods. Steer clear of daytime naps and vary their routine.

There are a number of online questionnaires available that will reveal your Ayurvedic type.

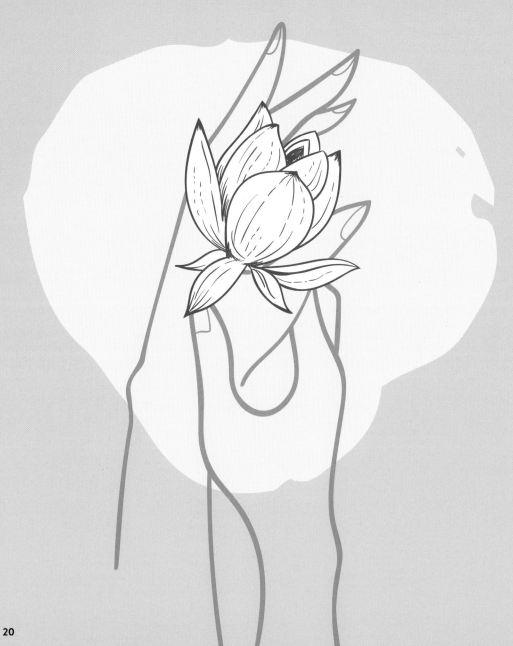

Reiki

Reiki is a Japanese healing practice that was founded in the early twentieth century. The word "reiki" is a combination of two Japanese words, *rei*, which means "God's wisdom" and *ki*, which means "life force energy". It works by channelling the unseen life force that flows through everything. During a session, a reiki practitioner will place their hands lightly above or on your body to encourage healing.

You don't have to be religious or hold any particular beliefs in order to be able to channel this healing energy and while it is most common for practitioners to lay their hands on you, they can also practise reiki from a distance if you prefer.

You can give yourself a full reiki self-treatment at home, by laying your hands on one of your chakras – energy centres located on your body – for 3–5 minutes. As you do it, imagine you are channelling universal life force energy through your hands.

Here are the main chakras on your body:

- **Crown chakra** – gently place hands on or above your head.

- **Third eye chakra** – place your palms over your eyes.

- **Throat chakra** – hold your hands on either side of your throat.

- **Heart chakra** – place your palms over your chest in the heart area.

- **Solar plexus chakra** – put your hands, one above the other, on the area just below the breastbone.

- **Sacral chakra** – place your hands either side of the navel with your fingertips touching.

- **Root chakra** – hover your hands lightly over the groin area in a "V" shape.

Yoga

Yoga originated in ancient India more than 5,000 years ago and aims to harmonize the mind, body and spirit through a series of postures, breathing techniques, meditation and relaxation.

There are more than 100 different forms of yoga with a style to suit all ages and levels of ability.

Here are some of the most popular:

Iyengar – a gentle form of yoga that encourages you to move your body into alignment. Great for everyone.

Ashtanga – a dynamic practice that links breath to movements, done in quick sequences with continuous flow. Better suited to experienced yogis.

Kripalu – a slow and gentle form of yoga with considered body movements and an emphasis on cultivating a deeper mind/body awareness. Great for novices.

Hatha – one of the most commonly practised forms of yoga, which combines a series of gentle movements with controlled breathing. Perfect for beginners.

Bikram – also known as "hot yoga" – an intense practice that involves a series of challenging movements done in a room where the temperature is ramped up. Best for experienced yogis only.

Power – a fast-paced practice that improves body strength. Not suitable for beginners.

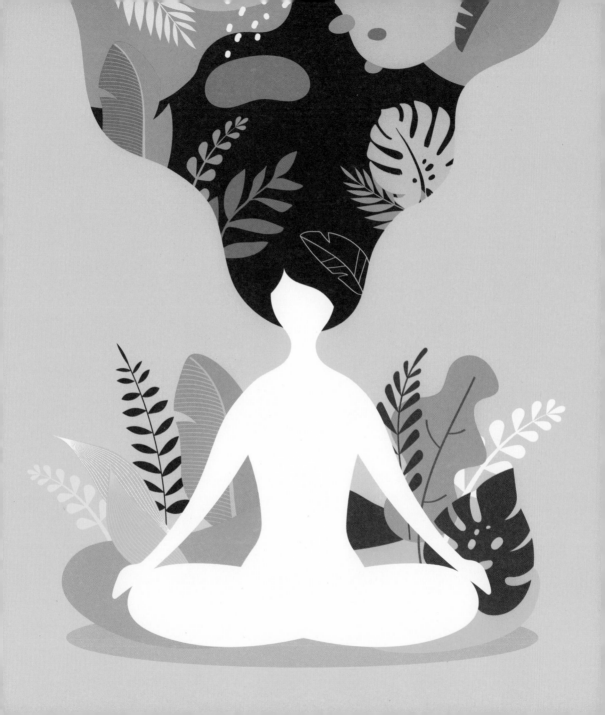

Yoga poses to try at home

If you'd like to give yoga a try, here are a few poses to start you off. Make sure you wear comfortable clothes and, if possible, use a yoga mat. If you enjoy them, why not look up a class near you, or try out some yoga apps or videos online?

Child's pose – ideal for stretching the lower back. Kneel down, sitting back on your heels with your knees slightly apart, then lean forward to rest your forehead on the mat and stretch your arms out in front of you. Rest here and breathe deeply. Try placing your arms at your sides for a gentler stretch.

Cat pose – gives the spine and stomach a gentle massage. Form a tabletop position on all fours with a flat back. As you exhale, round your back and gently tilt the crown of your head toward the floor. Hold for a few seconds and then, when you inhale, straighten your back.

Mountain pose – helps improve posture. Stand up straight with your feet together, tighten your belly, let your arms fall naturally by your side with palms facing upward and lengthen your neck. Feel strong as you take 5–10 slow breaths.

Downward dog – a good stretch for the lower back, hamstrings and calves. Kneel on all fours with your knees directly below your hips and hands slightly in front of your shoulders. Spread your fingers, exhale and lift your knees away from the floor so that your body forms a V shape. Lift your bottom toward the ceiling and draw your chest toward your thighs. Hold for several deep breaths.

Hero pose – great for posture. Sit back on your heels and bring your feet out to each side so they are either side of your hips, heels facing the ceiling. Place your hands palms down on top of your knees. Engage your abs, lengthen your neck, look ahead and take 10 gentle breaths.

Cobra – stretches the whole back. Lie face down with your toes flat on the floor and hands palms down next to the shoulders. Lift your upper torso by pressing the floor with both hands, keep your elbows close to your body, pull your shoulders back and engage your abs. Look ahead to ensure that your neck stays long. Hold for five breaths and repeat.

T'ai chi

T'ai chi is a Chinese martial art that was developed in the thirteenth century, but is now practised around the world to promote good physical and mental health. It consists of a series of gentle, flowing physical movements that are performed with a combination of breath work and mindfulness.

According to the principles of traditional Chinese medicine, t'ai chi movements help stimulate the vital flow of energy known as "chi" (also known as "qi", see page 15) in the body. Research indicates that t'ai chi improves balance, flexibility and posture, promotes healing and can even stave off dementia. It is beneficial for people with chronic illness and relieves stress.

Although it is a gentle, low-impact form of exercise, it strengthens the body and is particularly good for conditioning the core muscles of the back and abdomen. Due to the meditative nature of t'ai chi, it is also good for your mental and emotional health. You can either look for a class locally, try some online teaching or have a go at some of the beginner's videos on YouTube.

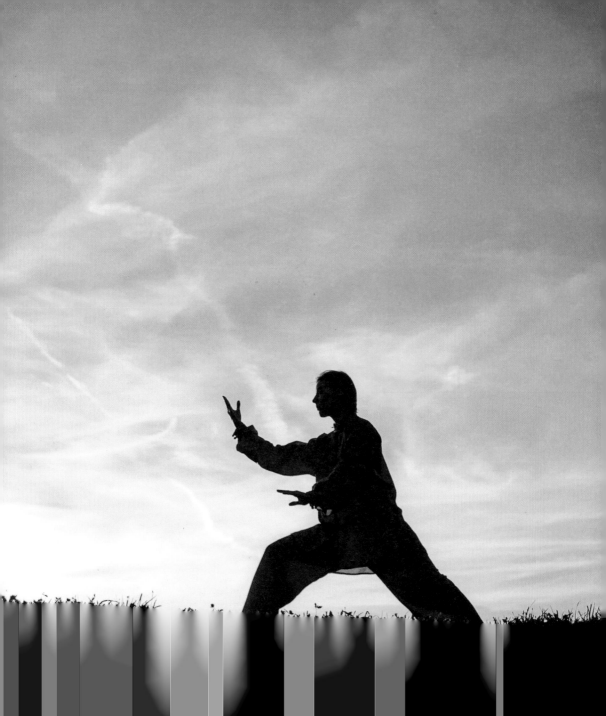

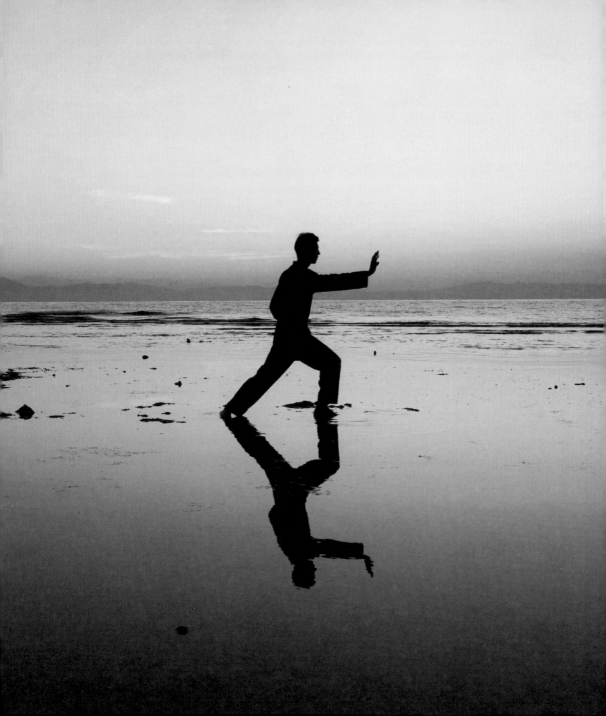

Qigong

Qigong comes under the umbrella of Chinese medicine and features gentle movements that are similar to those in t'ai chi. The purpose of qigong is to channel the vital life force that runs through everything in the universe with a mix of postures, breathing techniques, meditations and guided imagery. This is to ensure that this energy is free flowing with no blockages.

Once the movements are perfected with practice and patience, you learn how to bring meditation into them. The practice also shares similarities with yoga as many of the postures are held for long periods of time with a strong focus on breathing techniques and an awareness of body and mind.

Qigong strengthens the body, improves digestion, boosts the immune system, promotes healing and relieves stress. Experienced practitioners are able to radiate the "qi" or life force so that others can benefit from it.

There are three categories of qigong:

- **Medical qigong** – a slow workout performed with coordinated breath to improve health and well-being.

- **Meditation qigong** – a meditation that is carried out while sitting, standing or lying down for mind/body integration and emotional and spiritual well-being.

- **Martial qigong** – dynamic movements combined with deep long breaths used by martial artists to boost their prowess.

Medical and meditation qigong are ideal for beginners. There are plenty of videos available online and you can also find one-to-one classes on the internet.

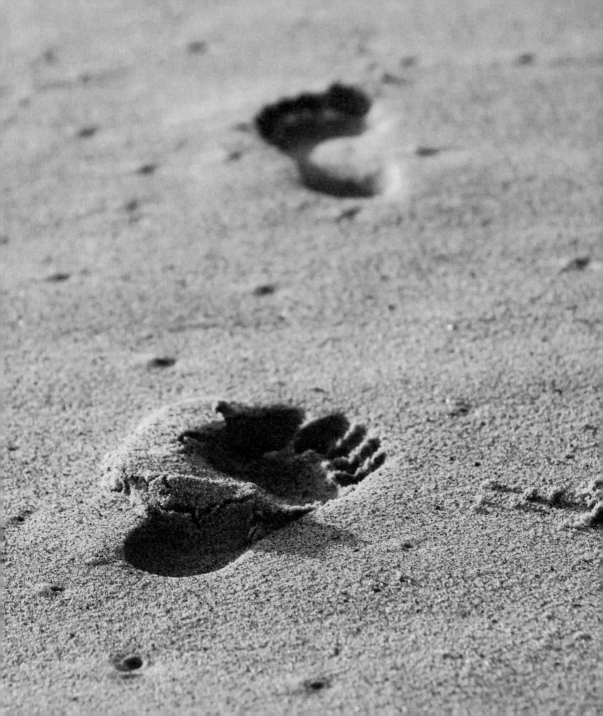

Reflexology

Reflexology is a touch therapy that uses points on the feet, hands and ears that correspond to other areas of the body. It is used to treat a range of conditions from stress and anxiety through to poor digestion, back pain and fertility issues. It dates back to ancient Egypt, India and China, but wasn't introduced into the West until the early twentieth century.

Reflexology aims to keep the "qi" energy flowing freely throughout the body. Using their fingertips, practitioners can work out where there are imbalances and apply pressure to the feet, hands and ears accordingly.

Reflexology at home

You can give yourself a reflexology massage in the comfort of your own home, while seated in a comfortable chair that allows easy access to the soles of your feet. Use a massage oil and an acupressure foot chart to help you locate the right pressure points. Here are a few to get started with: for back problems work on the heels, massage the arch of your foot for digestive issues and work on the fleshy area just below the little toe for sore shoulders. Press your thumb into the spot you've identified and knead the area for about 30 seconds. Move on to the next spot when you feel that any tension has been eased.

According to research, a 5-minute foot massage can reduce stress levels and blood pressure.

Cupping

Cupping dates back to ancient Chinese, Egyptian and Middle Eastern cultures. A cup (usually made from glass) is placed on the skin (usually on the back) and then a vacuum effect is created, either by heating the cup or using a hand-held suction pump. This causes the skin to be pulled upwards where it will redden as the blood vessels expand. Each cup is left in place for around 3 minutes.

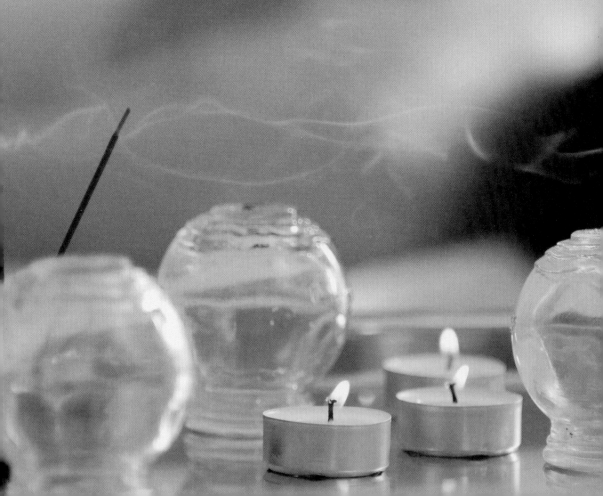

It is believed that the increased blood flow stimulated by cupping triggers healing, relieves muscle tension, improves circulation and reduces inflammation.

Cupping treatment can cause some soreness and temporary bruising that usually looks a lot worse than it feels – definitely not recommended if you are thinking of wearing anything backless! You'll find cupping practitioners based at most holistic healing centres or you can look online to find your local cupping society.

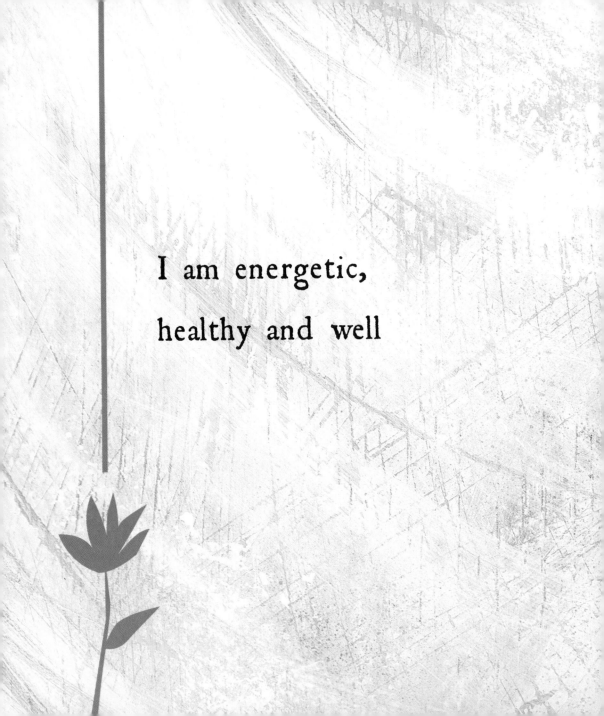

I am energetic,
healthy and well

Your body has natural healing capacities that nobody in the field of medicine can pretend ultimately to understand.

Wayne Dyer

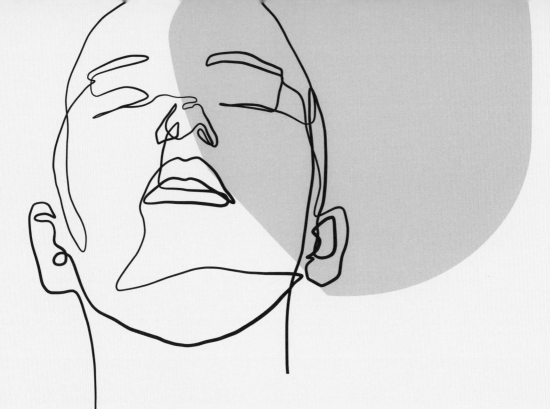

Hypnotherapy

Hypnotherapy uses hypnosis and the power of suggestion to change detrimental habits and treat any conditions that have an underlying mental cause. During the session, the therapist will gently guide you into a relaxed state, but you will still be awake and in control. While you are under hypnosis, the therapist will talk to your subconscious mind – that's the part of your mind that is responsible for automatically triggered feelings and emotions.

There are many different types of hypnotherapy and it is worth doing some research to find out which approach will best suit you. Here are some of the main branches of hypnotherapy:

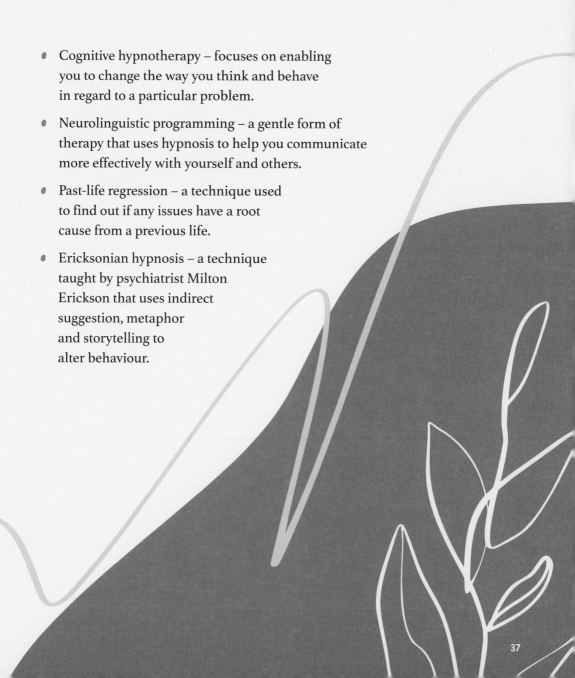

- Cognitive hypnotherapy – focuses on enabling you to change the way you think and behave in regard to a particular problem.

- Neurolinguistic programming – a gentle form of therapy that uses hypnosis to help you communicate more effectively with yourself and others.

- Past-life regression – a technique used to find out if any issues have a root cause from a previous life.

- Ericksonian hypnosis – a technique taught by psychiatrist Milton Erickson that uses indirect suggestion, metaphor and storytelling to alter behaviour.

Craniosacral therapy

Despite the name's suggestion, craniosacral therapy does not only involve working on the head – the practice is said to gently manipulate the bones of the skull, spine and pelvis so that the cerebrospinal fluid in the central nervous system can flow freely. It is thought to relieve any pressure in the head, neck or back and can be beneficial if you have problems in any of those areas. It is very gentle and all you can feel is the pressure of the therapist's hands on your body.

Treatment is done fully clothed and usually lasts for an hour. During this time, the therapist will lightly touch your head, spine and other areas of your body, encouraging relaxation and to trigger healing. Because it is non-invasive, it is suitable for everybody and patients often report feeling energized and more at peace after a session. It is recommended for general well-being and is reported to be beneficial in the treatment of depression, asthma, ADHD, pain, tension and back problems.

In order to benefit from craniosacral therapy, you may need more than one session. It works well in conjunction with other healing approaches such as yoga, acupuncture and hypnotherapy.

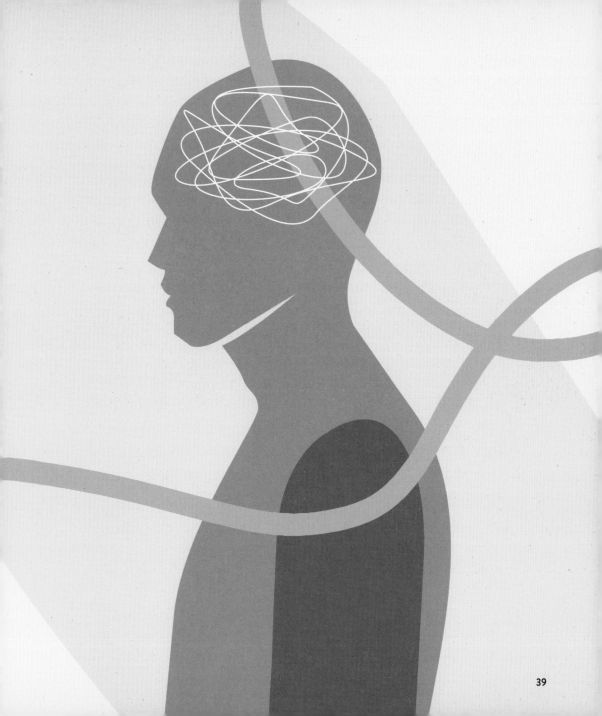

Chapter Two

Herbs and Natural Medicine

The miracle of nature is that it provides the nutrients and medicine needed to heal our bodies. Herbal medicine is plant based and suitable for people of all ages. Like all holistic healers, a herbalist or naturopath (a practitioner who believes in the body's ability to heal itself) will treat the whole person, and emotional well-being is just as important as physiology. Herbal medicines come in many forms, from fresh or dried herbs through to juices, powders, creams and poultices.

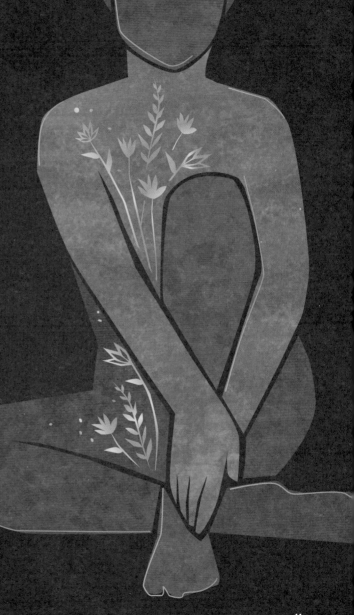

Mother Earth's medicine chest is full of healing herbs of incomparable worth.

Robin Rose Bennett

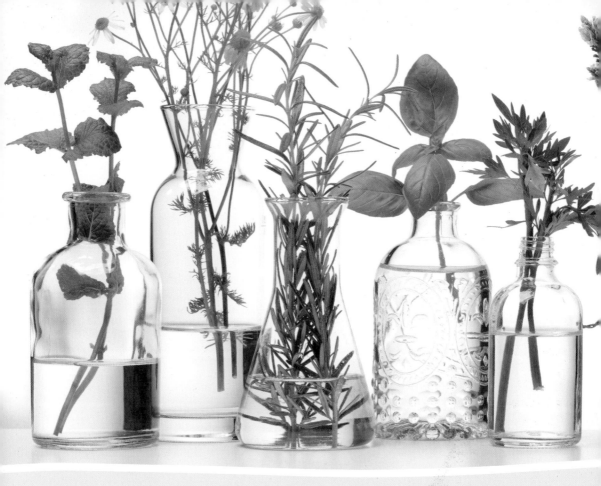

Why try natural medicine?

Natural medicine has been around for thousands of years and plant extracts are, in fact, contained in many of the medications made by the large pharmaceutical companies – the first statins (cholesterol-lowering medication) were all made from natural sources and there is even a dementia drug that contains an extract from daffodils.

Science has proven that many natural medicines are as effective as synthetic drugs, but choosing a natural alternative doesn't mean you have to turn your back on conventional

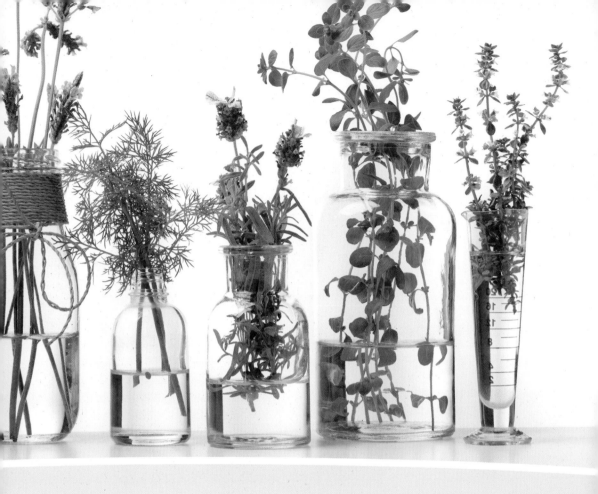

practice. As long as your GP or surgeon and natural health practitioner know what treatment you are having, the two can complement each other. You are also less likely to experience side effects with natural medicines and, as an added bonus, they are kind to the environment.

In a world where more people are concerned about what they are putting into their bodies, it makes sense to look for natural treatments where appropriate. Nature is clever and the plant world provides us with medicine for nearly all of our ailments.

Common herbs and their medicinal uses

Plants have been the basis of medical treatment for centuries. Here are some of the most popular.

Garlic – related to the onion, garlic has been used as a medicine for thousands of years for its antibiotic and antidepressant properties.

Aloe vera – known as "the wonder plant", aloe vera grows in North America and the sap is used to heal wounds, burns and other ailments. It is also said to ease constipation when taken orally.

Gingko – gingko biloba is a tree native to China and extract from its leaves is supposedly useful in the treatment of asthma, bronchitis and fatigue. It is also said to improve circulation.

Clove – used by cooks as a flavouring, cloves can also soothe toothaches and upset stomachs.

Liquorice root – liquorice is a flowering plant that belongs to the bean family and extract from its root has been used for centuries to treat ailments like stomach ulcers, infections and bronchitis.

Arnica – this plant that grows mainly in Siberia and central Europe is used as an anti-inflammatory.

Ginger – used by cooks and sold as a herbal supplement, ginger relieves nausea, helps prevent morning sickness and eases the symptoms of colds and flu.

Lavender – aside from its heavenly scent, lavender has been used for centuries as an antiseptic. It also aids sleep when used in the form of an essential oil dabbed on to the pillow.

Camomile – these daisy-like plants are dried and consumed as a tea. Camomile is used by herbalists to treat anxiety, insomnia and tummy upsets.

Thyme – the flowers, leaves and oil of this herb are used to treat colds, infections, burns and period pains.

St John's wort – this flowering plant is a powerful antidepressant and is also used to ease insomnia.

Peppermint – one of the oldest known herbs to be used for its medicinal properties, peppermint is used for the treatment of nausea, indigestion and cold symptoms.

Turmeric – a bright-yellow spice that has been used for thousands of years as a powerful anti-inflammatory. It also supports the joints and eases indigestion..

It is always best to seek advice if you intend to take herbs to treat an illness. You can find a trained practitioner from your local holistic healing clinic or the national register for professional herbalists.

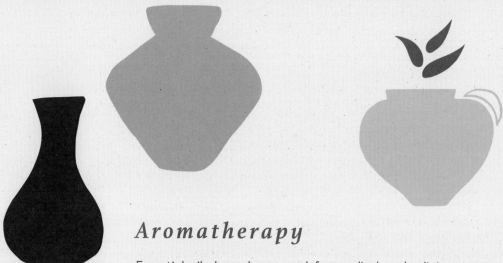

Aromatherapy

Essential oils have been used for medical and religious purposes for thousands of years, but the term "aromatherapy" wasn't coined until the early twentieth century when a French doctor called René-Maurice Gattefossé discovered the antiseptic benefits of lavender when treating a burn. His later work showed that essential oils were beneficial in the healing of other types of wound too.

Aromatherapy is based on the use of aromatic essential oils to lift and heal mind, body and spirit through skin absorption and sense of smell. You can use the oils in diffusers, lotions, bath salts and spritzers, or by putting a few drops on your pillow or a clean handkerchief, but the most glorious way of benefitting from their heavenly smells and healing properties is through massage.

Each oil has a set of properties, uses and effects and there will be a perfect blend to suit you. You can reap the rewards of DIY aromatherapy at home or find a trained aromatherapist who will devise a bespoke treatment plan to meet your needs. The oils themselves are concentrated and should not be applied to the skin unless they are mixed with a base oil, such as sweet almond.

Some of the most powerful essential oils and their benefits:

Orange – cleansing, purifying and stimulating.

Rosemary – respiratory support, aids memory, digestion and healthy hair.

Tea tree – cleansing, boosts skin health and immunity.

Lavender – calming, antiseptic and helps with stress relief.

Rose – boosts emotional balance, clears skin.

Jasmine – mood-balancing.

Frankincense – aids emotional support and skin health.

Basil – soothes menstrual problems and sore muscles, as well as boosting mental alertness.

Vetiver – calming and immune-boosting.

Marjoram – enhances heart and muscle health.

Lime – detoxifying and stimulating.

Dill – improves digestion.

Bach flower remedies

Dr Edward Bach (1886–1936) was a surgeon and bacteriologist who conducted research into the field of immunology. He concluded that any illness caused by negative emotions such as stress or fear could be alleviated using essences distilled from a range of 38 different wild flowers. He said: "Healing with the clean, pure, beautiful agents of nature is surely the one method of all, which appeals to most of us."

Each of the 38 essences has qualities that correspond to a particular set of emotions. They are 100 per cent natural and work by helping to rebalance thoughts and feelings to restore equilibrium. Flower essence is made by placing flowers in water and creating an infusion by exposing them to a heat source. The flowers themselves are discarded and the liquid is preserved (usually with alcohol), diluted and stored.

The treatment works on the basis that plants have a particular vibrational frequency that resonates with certain thoughts, feelings or emotions There is no scientific evidence to back up this claim, but many people swear by it.

Today, Bach flower remedies are available from most health food shops and come in various forms including drops, sprays, creams, pastilles, pearls and lozenges. They are safe to be used by anyone, including babies and even pets and plants. There are no side effects and you cannot overdose.

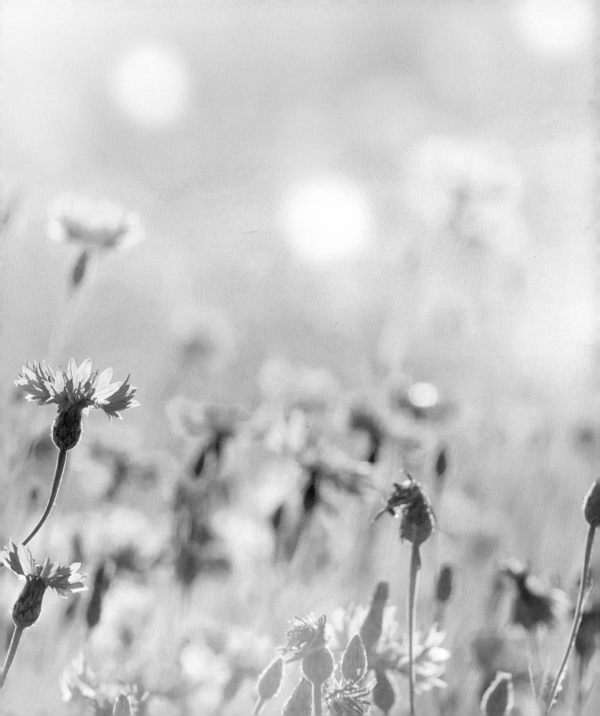

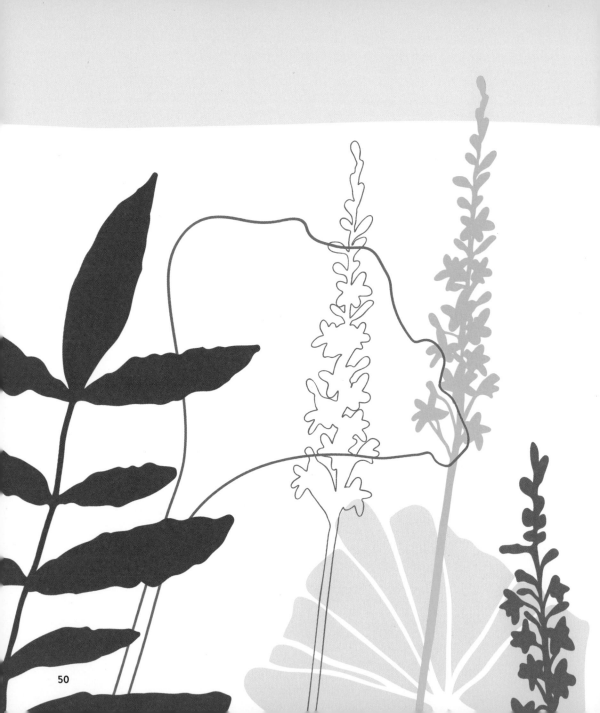

The flower essences

Ten flower essences and the negative emotions they are said to dispel:

- **Agrimony** – this essence restores a person's ability to express their true feelings and is said to help with addiction, anxiety and insomnia. Bach said it was useful for those who "are tormented and restless and worried in mind or body".

- **Beech** – helps those who are naturally critical, judgemental and intolerant. Bach described the essence as something for "those who feel the need to see more good and beauty in all that surrounds them".

- **Chestnut bud** – beneficial for those who tend to make the same mistakes again and again without learning. Chestnut bud is said to encourage the wisdom needed to move forward in life in a more positive way.

- **Elm** – those who need this essence find themselves taking on too much and risking burnout. They may also have an inclination toward depression and exhaustion.

- **Holly** – the predominant quality of holly is love, and this essence is for those who want to open their hearts and rid themselves of envy, jealousy and hatred.

- **Hornbeam** – if you're stuck in a boring routine or pattern, feel tired all the time and lack mental clarity, hornbeam could be the answer.

- **Pine** – for anyone who finds themselves saying "sorry" all the time and suffers from feelings of guilt, shame and unworthiness.

- **Scleranthus** – gives you the mental strength to make firm decisions.

- **Walnut** – helps to ease negative emotions linked to menopause and puberty and also to help you let go of the old in order to embrace the new.

- **Willow** – helps to ease resentment and bitterness and restores the quality of forgiveness.

Nature supports,
loves and
nourishes me

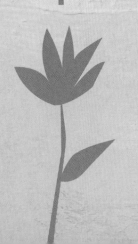

Look deep into nature
and you will understand
everything better.

Albert Einstein

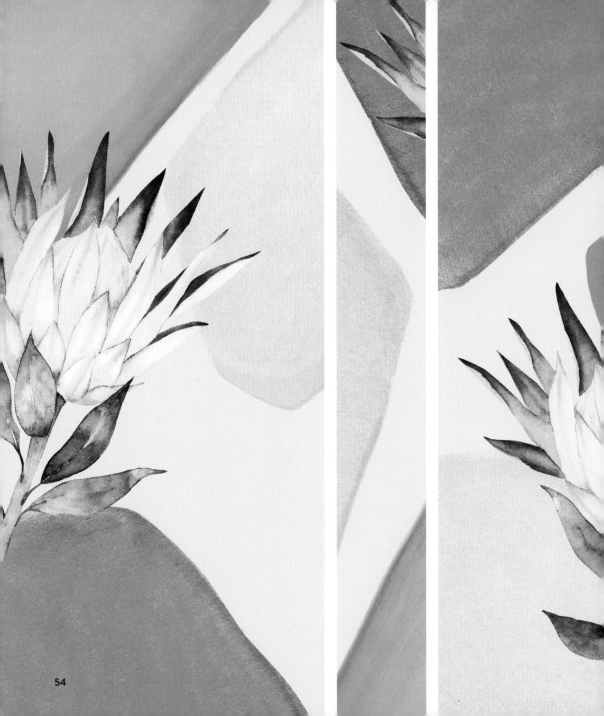

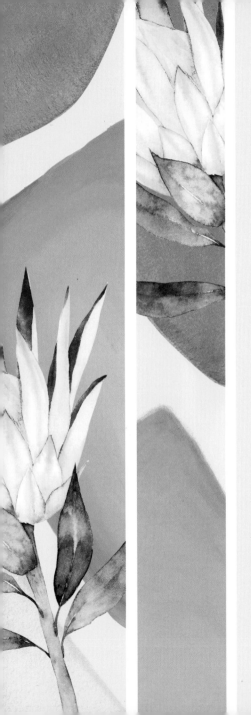

Rescue Remedy

Rescue Remedy is a mix of five Bach flower essences in one dose, blended to deal with emotional crises from exam nerves through to accidents and dealing with bad news. Many people carry Rescue Remedy with them just in case.

It is taken orally, whenever the need arises, and can be ingested in various forms from pastilles and sprays through to lozenges and drops. Rescue Remedy is not habit-forming and there are no side effects.

The five essences in Rescue Remedy are:

- **Impatiens** – alleviates impatience and lowers stress. It also encourages you to slow down in both thought and action.

- **Star of Bethlehem** – helps ease trauma and shock, and stops the resultant negative emotions from holding you back. It will also make you feel stronger.

- **Cherry plum** – stops you from feeling out of control, helps to instil a feeling of calm and enables you to think more clearly.

- **Rock rose** – relieves panic and terror, and encourages mental clarity and courage.

- **Clematis** – brings clarity and present-moment awareness to a situation.

Food as medicine

While it is widely known that a healthy diet will help protect your body from disease, many foods have medicinal effects that can treat illness and manage chronic disease. Thanks to nutritional science, we know more about the healing effects of food than ever before.

Try incorporating the following foods into your diet on a regular basis and see if you notice a difference:

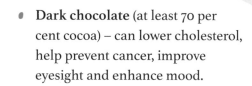

- **Dark chocolate** (at least 70 per cent cocoa) – can lower cholesterol, help prevent cancer, improve eyesight and enhance mood.

- **Bananas** – help to ease anxiety.

- **Blueberries** – good for a healthy heart and immune system and for treating urinary problems.

- **Broccoli** – said to reduce the risk of cancer.

- **Salmon** – fights inflammation and protects against heart disease.

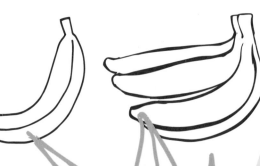

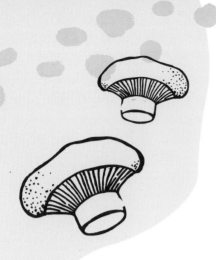

- **Mushrooms** – a good source of vitamin D, which is said to inhibit the growth of tumours and be beneficial for Alzheimer's.

- **Walnuts** – mood-boosting and they contribute to memory function.

- **Coffee** – rich in antioxidants, which fight inflammation and help stop tooth decay.

- **Yogurt** – good for bones and a healthy gut.

- **Avocado** – improves good fats in the blood, which can reduce the risk of heart disease and stroke.

- **Sauerkraut** (raw fermented cabbage) – combats digestive problems and inflammation, and may reduce the risk of depression and Alzheimer's.

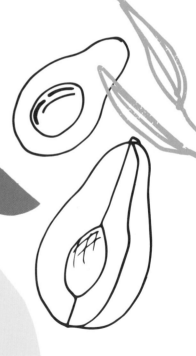

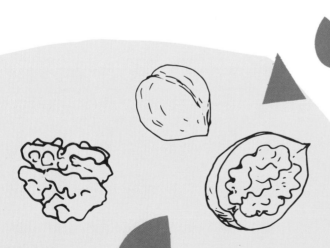

Sleep

Getting at least 7–9 hours of sleep each night is essential for good health and while there are remedies available, it is always best to aid sleep naturally.

Try these simple tips to ensure you get enough shut-eye:

- Don't look at a screen for at least 2 hours before you go to bed; keep phones, laptops, etc. out of the bedroom.

- If you must stare at a screen in the evening, use a blue-light-filtering app.

- Sleep in complete darkness – if you can, invest in blackout blinds, heavy curtains or a sleep mask.

- Stay cool – the room should be between 16–20°C (60–68°F).

- Go to bed and wake up at the same time each day so your body gets used to a routine.

- Avoid coffee, tea and alcohol for several hours (the longer the better) before going to bed.

- Sprinkle a few drops of lavender oil on your pillow.

- Make sure you are getting enough vitamin B6 – adults need 1.3mg a day and a lack of it causes cracks at the corner of the mouth, scaly lips and itchy rashes. It is found in cheese, fish, lentils, spinach, avocadoes and sunflower seeds.

- Have a cup of camomile tea before bedtime.

- Try some yoga nidra, or yogic sleep – a yoga practice that achieves a meditative state.

- Take magnesium, either as tablets or topically. The right levels of magnesium in the body make it easier to fall asleep.

- Exercise during the day for at least 30 minutes, five to six times a week.

- Turn your clock to face the other way to stop you worrying about how many hours of sleep you have left.

- Keep a pad and pen by the bed so you can write down any thoughts that are whirring through your mind and stopping you from getting to sleep.

Chapter Three

Crystal Healing

Crystals are formed underground and their appearance depends very much on the growing conditions of their environment. While there is no scientific evidence to support the use of crystals as a healing tool, they have been used for centuries by ancient cultures as a cure for illness and are still popular to this day. People who use them swear by their powers and, thanks to their beauty, they are lovely objects to have around the home.

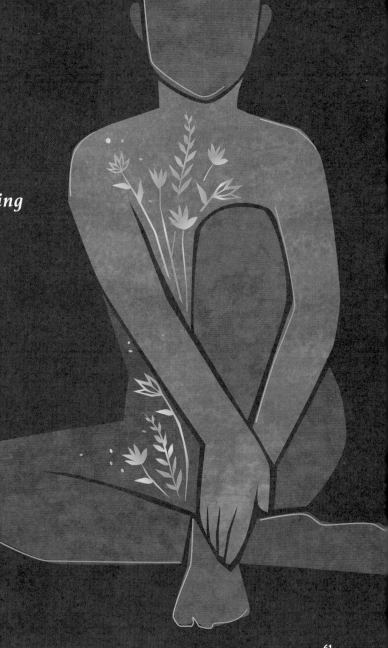

*Crystals are living
beings at the beginning
of creation.*

Nikola Tesla

Crystal healing

Crystals have been used as a tool for healing for centuries. The ancient Egyptians used rose quartz to eradicate wrinkles, and Romans and Greeks once thought that amethyst would prevent them from getting drunk.

Different types of crystal are thought to have their own unique energies, and it is believed they can heal physical, emotional and spiritual aspects of ourselves.

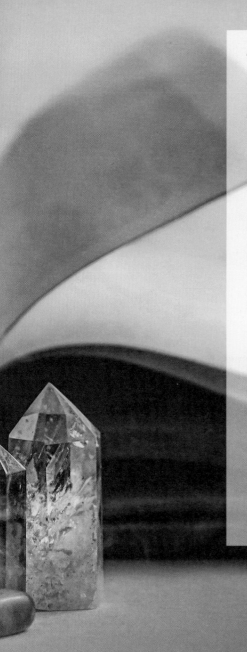

The top 10 crystals used for healing and their spiritual associations

- **Amethyst** – peace, healing and intuition.
- **Rose quartz** – forgiveness, love and self-esteem.
- **Tiger's eye** – courage, clarity and strength.
- **Hematite** – grounding, anxiety relief and memory.
- **Emerald** – hope, renewal and friendship.
- **Citrine** – happiness, abundance and vision.
- **Celestite** – spirituality, prosperity and dreaming.
- **Turquoise** – luck, balance and the immune system.
- **Desert rose** – motivation, energy and harmony.
- **Jasper** – stress easing and dispelling of negative vibes.

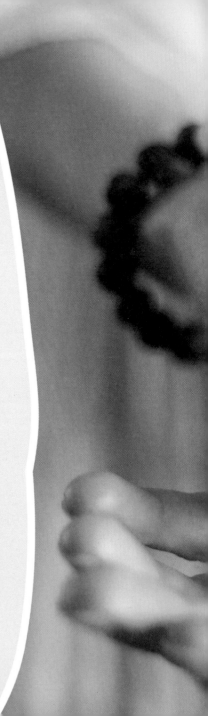

How to heal yourself with crystals

First, you need to find the right stone. Each variety has its own special properties, so pick one that is in line with your needs. Holding it in your hand, close your eyes, take a few deep breaths and clasp it tightly. If you feel sensations such as heat, cold, tingling, peacefulness and love, then it's a sign that you have found the right crystal.

Now you've found your stone, you need to let it know exactly what you would like to receive. Hold your crystal as you meditate and when your mind is quiet, ask it to clear itself of any unwanted energy and then tell it what you wish for. Be sure to say thank you afterwards.

Once you have booted up your crystal, you can either carry it with you throughout the day, hold it while meditating, pop it in the bathtub while you enjoy a soak or place it on a specific chakra with the aim of encouraging the invisible life force energy to flow freely – see page 68 for more on the power of chakras.

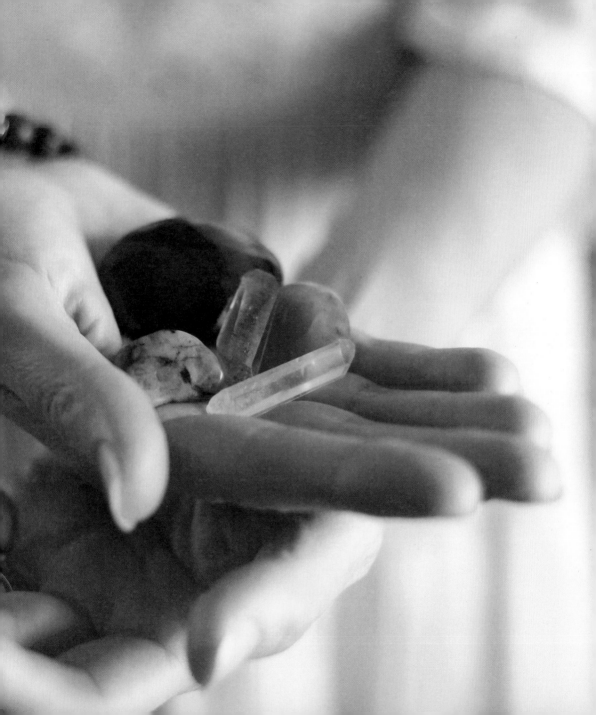

Create harmony in the home with crystals

Because they are so eye-catching, crystals are ideal for use in the home. As well as having your favourite small crystals to carry with you at all times, you can also buy large crystals that will double as beautiful ornaments as well as acting as powerful tools for creating positive energy indoors.

If you meditate or practise yoga in a particular room, it's a nice idea to create a mini altar. Crystal expert Heather Askinosie suggests that you place some on a piece of paper that has your healing intention written on it.

When selecting which crystal you want to place in a room, think of the quality of energy that you want to suffuse the space with. Askinosie suggests that you cleanse your home with a sage stick before you bring crystals in, to shift any negative energy that's hanging around.

Here are five crystals that are perfect for the home:

- **Blue lace agate** – a calming crystal that is ideal for bringing a sense of peace to your bedroom.

- **Desert rose** – a pretty, clear stone that will fill your home with uplifting energy.

- **Carnelian** – a vibrant crystal that is good for inspiring creativity. Great for the kitchen or a home office.

- **Black tourmaline** – a useful tool if you want to block the entry of negative energy. Many choose to have it by the front door.

- **Amethyst** – with its powers to assist with clear thinking and focus, a selection of amethyst crystals is perfect to have on your desk.

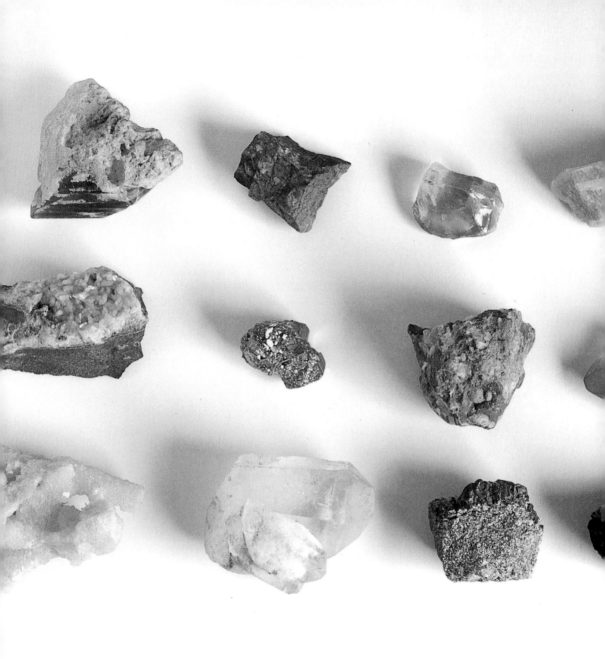

What are chakras?

Chakras are energy centres that run down the middle of our bodies, from the crown of the head, down to the base of the spine. There are seven of them and each has an associated colour, which reflects its vibrational frequency. Chakras date back to early Hindu and Buddhist traditions, and are at the root of many forms of holistic healing including yoga, reiki, acupuncture, acupressure and pranic healing.

The word *chakra* means "wheel" in Sanskrit and each chakra can be seen as a spinning wheel of energy; this energy is known as prana. As prana is in a constant state of flow, it is essential that the chakras remain open. If they get blocked or spin too slowly, then well-being suffers.

The chakras correspond to different organs as well as overall physical, emotional and spiritual health. It only takes one chakra to be out of alignment for the whole body to be pushed out of balance.

There is no need to panic if a practitioner tells you that one or some of your chakras are blocked, because it is a temporary state and healthy movement can be restored using a variety of techniques. You can do it yourself at home using meditation, stretching, breathing exercises and visualizations.

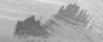

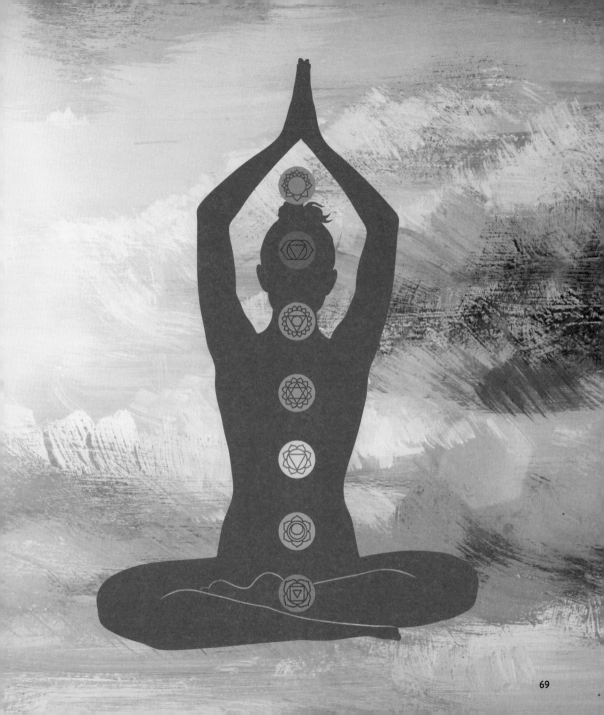

The seven chakras

Chakra	Position	Colour	Sense	Powers	How to unblock
Root chakra	At the base of the spine	Red	Smell	Regulates instinct, survival and security	Walking in nature or practising yoga
Sacral chakra	Just below the navel	Orange	Touch and taste	Regulates creativity, sociability and sexuality	Pampering yourself
Solar plexus chakra	In the stomach region	Yellow	Sight	Regulates mental health, confidence and vitality	Trusting your gut instincts
Heart chakra	In the chest	Green	Touch	Regulates balance, compassion and prosperity	Doing something for others

Chakra	Position	Colour	Sense	Powers	How to unblock
Throat chakra	In the throat	Blue	Listening	Regulates self-expression, trust and speech	Speaking your mind
Third eye chakra	In the middle of your forehead, just above the eyebrows	Indigo	Intuition	Regulates imagination, psychic abilities and clarity	Meditating
Crown chakra	The top of the head	Violet	Knowing	Regulates spiritual connection, knowledge and enlightenment	Imagine white energy pouring into you from the crown

Chapter Four

Sensory Therapies

Our senses are inextricably linked with our health – what we see, hear, touch, smell and taste has an effect on our emotional well-being, which in turn influences our physical health. We constantly take in an impression of the world with our senses, and it is possible to use them in order to achieve balance and healing.

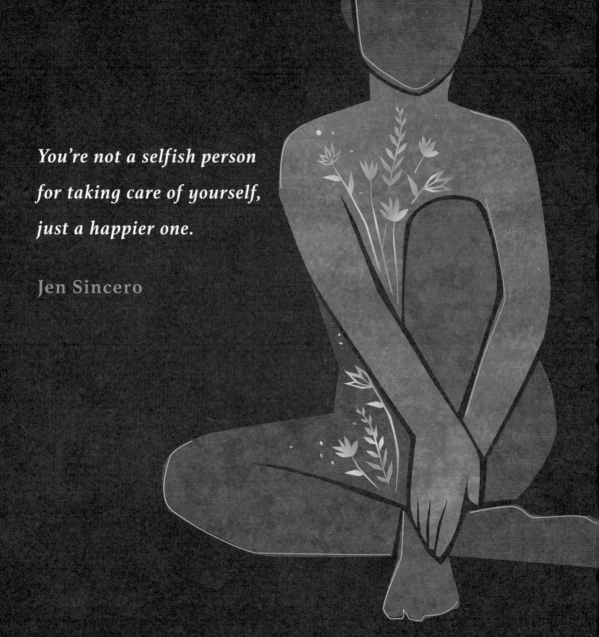

You're not a selfish person for taking care of yourself, just a happier one.

Jen Sincero

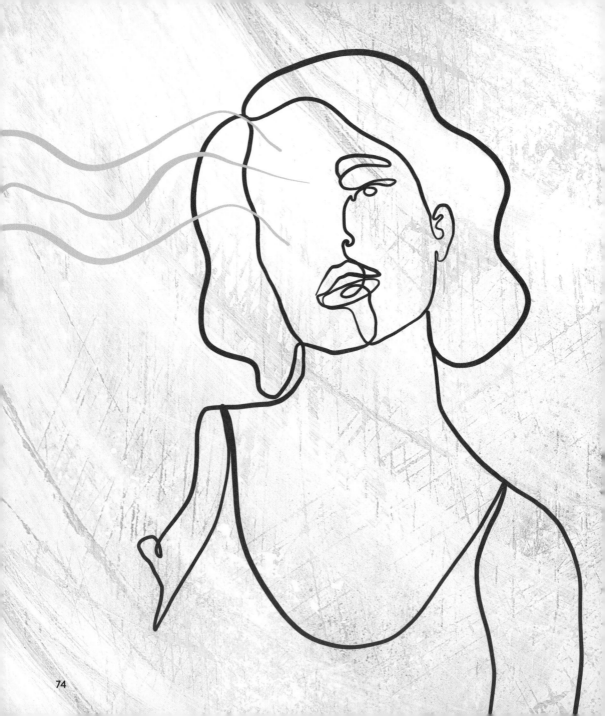

Sound as a healing tool

There is no disputing the therapeutic effects of sound. Most of us will have experienced it for ourselves, with certain songs or types of music that instantly make us feel better about life. In ancient Greece, music was used to cure mental health issues, and for centuries sound has been used by various cultures as a healing tool.

So how does it work? Sound travels in waves that pass through air, water, solid objects and all living things, including people. The human body is 75 per cent water, which makes it a good conductor for sound vibration. Healers believe that certain instruments (including the voice) create sounds that vibrate at frequencies that interact with the human energy field and release blockages. It is said that sound healing can lower stress, improve mood, lower blood pressure and cholesterol, improve sleep and even alter brainwaves for a more restful mind. The therapies on the next few pages all tap into this powerful tool.

Gong baths

Gong bathing is recommended for relaxation, stress relief, fatigue, anger, loneliness and for the relief of many other negative feelings that interfere with the body's equilibrium. There's no need to strip off for a gong bath; it is a relaxing, fully clothed experience where you lie down and literally bathe in the powerful sound waves created by gongs. Practitioners usually utilize several gongs, which between them can produce a broad range of tones. As the sound waves merge, the noise produced is otherworldly, powerful and embracing.

The sounds of the gongs encourage the mind to relax so that you can rest in a meditative state. It's important that you are warm and comfortable, so that you can relax deeply during the experience.

At first, the gongs are played very softly and the volume is increased gradually. There is no fixed rhythm, so your mind won't be able to follow a pattern. If you surrender and allow yourself to be consumed by the sound waves, you can enter a dreamlike and deeply meditative state that will leave you feeling invigorated at the end of the session.

Practitioners usually end the therapy by playing gentle bells, wind chimes or rattles, which help to ground you.

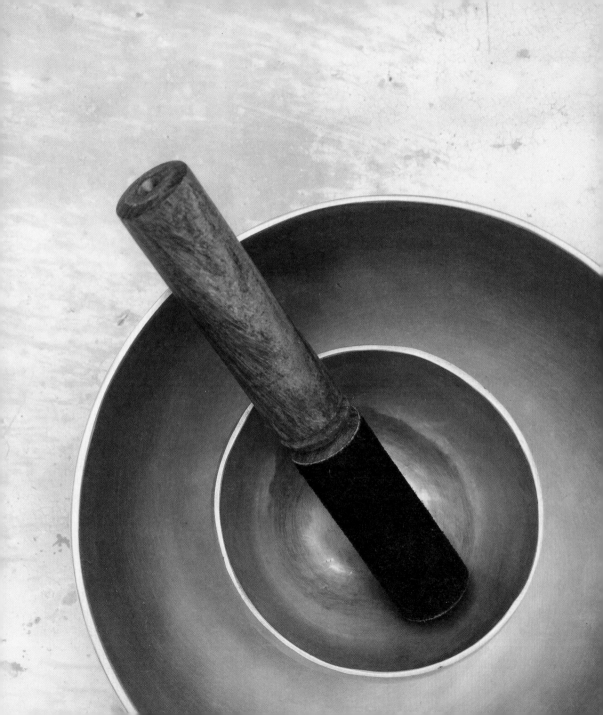

Chanting – Gregorian and kirtan

The act of chanting words and sounds can be incredibly soothing. Back in the ninth century, men and boys developed a method of singing Latin that inspired feelings of balance, tranquillity and a connection to God. It's called Gregorian chanting and it has barely changed since the Middle Ages. Its unique form and tonal quality means it is unlike any other form of music or song.

The Hindu tradition has its own form of chanting, called kirtan, which has become hugely popular in the West. It involves the singing or chanting of sacred mantras that praise the divine and often feature the names of gods and goddesses central to Hinduism and Sikhism. It's not a religious practice and anyone can do it. The ultimate aim is to awaken the love, joy and present-moment awareness within and because singing the words requires focus, kirtan helps bring the wandering mind back to the present moment. As well as soothing an overactive mind, kirtan energizes the body, helps shift emotional blockages and relieves stress.

During a session, the kirtan leader sings a mantra and the participants repeat it. You can also do this at home with pre-recorded kirtan music – there are lots of videos available on YouTube. Instructors will often play musical instruments such as a harmonium, drum or guitar. There are no rules. It doesn't matter if you can't hold a note and it's fine if you fancy getting up to dance, clap or even play a musical instrument of your own.

I let go of all my
negative thoughts and
embrace forgiveness,
love and positivity

Do you know that our soul
is composed of harmony?

Leonardo da Vinci

Taste therapy

What we taste in our mouths can have a huge effect on our emotions – you only need to pop a piece of chocolate on your tongue to know that. According to the Ayurvedic tradition, which originated in India, there are six categories of taste and each has an impact on our emotional and physical well-being.

The six tastes, or rasas as they are known, should all be present in any one meal as this will leave you feeling more satisfied, energized and less likely to snack. The tastes are:

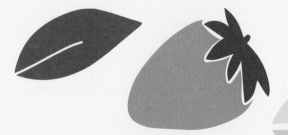

Sweet

Sweetness is grounding and nourishing when consumed in moderation. Rather than choosing confectionery, try to get your sugar intake from natural foods like dairy, wheat, dates and maple syrup.

Sour

Sourness stimulates the appetite, increases production of saliva and is thought to aid digestion. Lemons, pickles and vinegars are a good choice.

Salty

While too much salt is bad for you, it is vital for health and stimulates digestion. Try black olives, sea salt and tamari.

Pungent

Pungent foods clear the sinuses and speed up reactions. Go for hot peppers, ginger, mustard and garlic.

Bitter

Bitter tastes detoxify and lighten the mood. Raw green vegetables, turmeric and herbal teas are a good choice.

Astringent

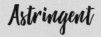

Astringent foods are purifying and strengthening. Bananas, pomegranates, green beans and okra fall into this category.

Colour therapy

The roots of colour therapy go back to 1550 BC. In ancient Egypt, Greece and China, rooms were painted in different colours in an attempt to cure various ailments. The practice was largely forgotten, but in 1810 Johann Wolfgang von Goethe, a writer, scientist and botanist, published *The Theory of Colour*, listing the therapeutic effect of each of the seven colours of the rainbow in treating physical and emotional problems, and revitalizing interest in the topic. The goal of colour treatment is to correct imbalances in the body's energy field, and as colour is comprised of light waves, each one has its own vibrational frequency.

You've probably already experienced the effects that colour can have on us. Yellow can feel like a joyous and uplifting shade, while green is calming and red is used to denote passion or anger, hence the phrase "seeing red".

Colour therapists treat patients in several ways. They either encourage you to look at the colours, drape different shades of silk on the skin or shine light at various points on the body.

Treatment usually begins and ends with green as it is the most balancing of colours.

You can use colour at home, too, either by choosing certain colours to wear or decorating rooms in shades that spark healing emotional responses. There's no need to paint an entire room – one orange wall in a kitchen or bathroom for example, may be enough to make you feel energized and clear headed.

The healing colour spectrum

Colours and their qualities:

Red – encourages vitality, stamina and passion.

Orange – associated with optimism, pleasure and sexuality.

Yellow – inspires and encourages feelings of happiness.

Green – the most balancing of colours, can improve your mood.

Blue – promotes feelings of peace and relaxation.

Indigo – allows you to view things from a higher perspective.

Violet – sparks intuition, imagination and creativity.

Guided imagery

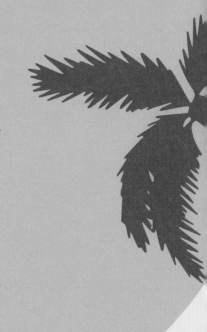

Guided imagery is a healing technique that involves picturing images in your mind that trigger a positive response. It is more than just a visual exercise as all the senses are involved and it is experienced throughout the whole body. The key to guided imagery is that if you can fully imagine seeing and feeling something, you can become it.

Studies have indicated that guided imagery meditation can reduce stress, lower blood pressure and ease pain. It is also a useful tool for anyone who is undergoing difficult medical procedures such as chemotherapy or dialysis.

It differs from hypnosis because you are using the power of your imagination to fire all the senses and immerse yourself in an altered state of mind.

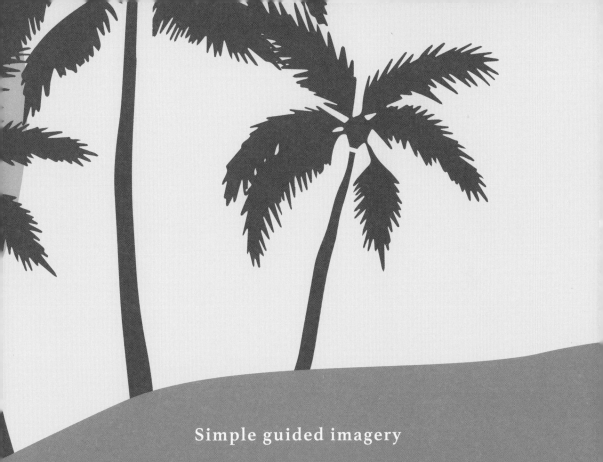

Simple guided imagery

1. Close your eyes and visualize a memory that makes you feel good. Picture the scene in as much detail as you can: imagine the sounds and smells and the temperature of the room, and the mood you experienced at the time. Notice any changes in how you feel as you fall deeper into the picture.

2. Practise this technique and, when you feel ready, apply it to life situations. You can picture a relaxing scene in times of stress or focus on something specific. For example, if you are about to give a talk in public, picture getting a round of applause at the end of it. If you have aches or pains, try to imagine them healing miraculously of their own accord.

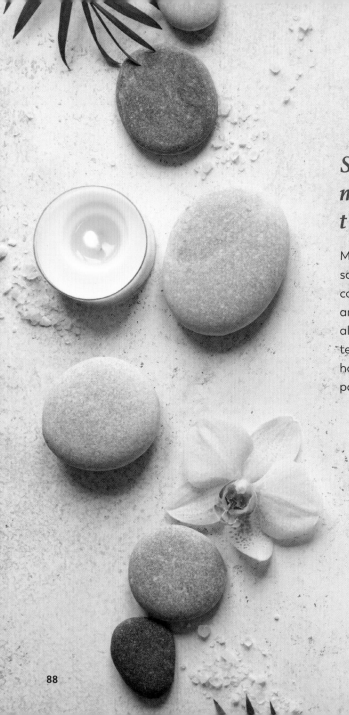

Simple massage techniques

Massage is wonderfully soothing, and while there are countless brilliant therapists around the world there are also some simple self-care techniques you can use at home to trigger muscle release, pain relief and relaxation.

Head

1. Place your thumbs on your cheekbone and your forefingers on your temples; apply gentle pressure in a circular motion to your temples with your fingers.

2. Without moving your thumbs, make circles along your brow until your fingertips meet. Do this for a few minutes. You can use scented oils for maximum pleasure.

Neck

1. Put your fingertips on the back of your neck where it meets the shoulders.

2. Apply firm pressure and hold for 20 seconds.

3. When you release your fingers, the muscle should feel more relaxed.

4. Roll your shoulders and repeat a few times.

Lower back

1. Take a tennis ball and position it between your lower back and the wall.

2. Move your body against the ball, applying comfortable pressure when you find areas of tension.

Flotation tank

Flotation tanks were first used in 1954 to test the effects of sensory deprivation and the first commercial tanks were used in 1972 to enable people to relax free from sensory input.

When you go for a float, you usually wear a bathing suit and enter a special water-filled tank containing Epsom salts, which allow you to float effortlessly. The water is usually up to 10 in. deep, and at a temperature that matches your skin. The tank is usually dark and silent – although you can switch on the light or listen to music if you prefer.

Floating in this environment allows your body and mind to drift into a state of deep relaxation. It is usually done for an hour at a time and is a great stress reliever as well as an aid to better sleep. There are numerous companies that offer flotation tank experiences and you can either pay for one float, or several sessions. If you want to try it at home, run a warm bath, add one to two cups of Epsom salts (flotation tanks are filled with 400–450 kg of Epsom salts, which enables you to float unaided!) and enjoy a soak by candlelight. It won't be quite the same as a flotation tank, but it will trigger a soothing natural relaxation response.

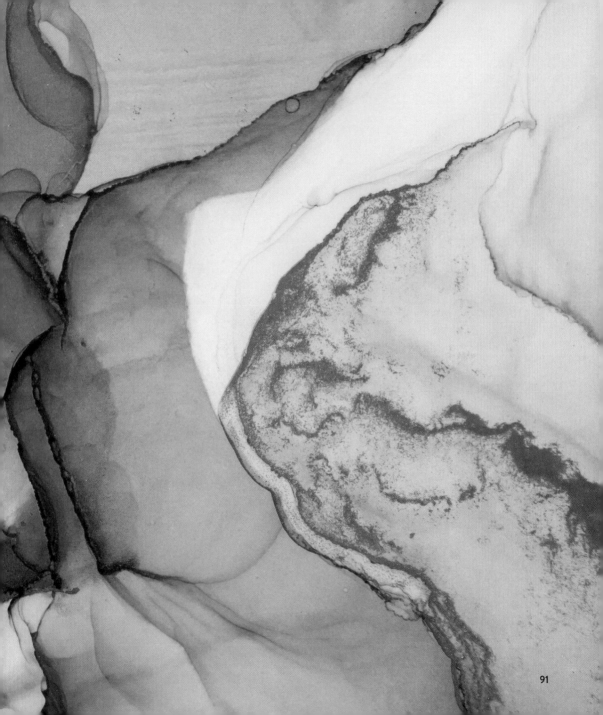

Chapter Five

The Power of Meditation

Have you noticed that meditation seems to be the new rock 'n' roll these days? Everyone is doing it, but actually, the practice has been around for thousands of years. It comes from the Latin word *meditatum*, which means "to ponder". While you can attend workshops and courses on the topic, meditation is really just the act of taking time out to do nothing, to ponder. You don't need a guru or a teacher and contrary to popular belief, it isn't even necessary to close your eyes. All that's required is a willingness to give it a go.

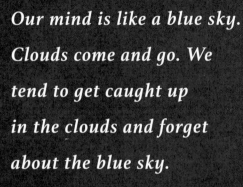

Our mind is like a blue sky. Clouds come and go. We tend to get caught up in the clouds and forget about the blue sky.

Andy Puddicombe

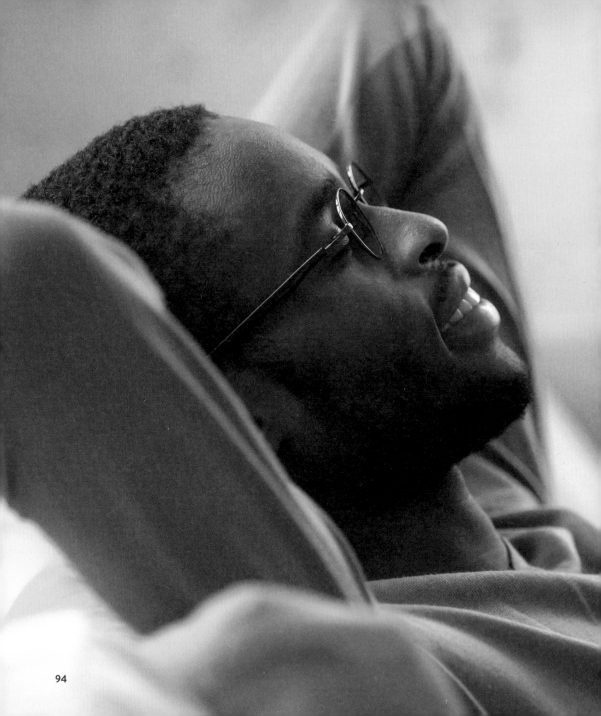

What is meditation?

Meditation is an exercise in training the busy mind to become more at ease. It is not about experiencing a feeling of bliss (although that can happen) or stopping your thoughts, and it doesn't involve intense concentration. Forget the pictures you've seen of people meditating on top of mountains looking serene – you may feel like this at times, but every meditation is different and no two sessions are the same. Anybody can do it and there is no such thing as a pass or fail.

Just like any form of exercise, it takes time and practice to master your mind – you wouldn't expect to achieve the perfect physique after a few visits to the gym and perseverance is key. It has a cumulative effect, so if you set aside time to do it daily, you will see results: regular meditators feel increased levels of inner peace, clarity, contentment and self-love. They also feel a deeper sense of connection to all other living things and experience more positive emotions such as joy, happiness and compassion.

When you meditate, you are taking time out to be alone with your mind and to get to know it. You are sitting with yourself. It really is that simple.

How to meditate

You can meditate for however long you like, but if you are a beginner, try starting with 10 minutes. Do it daily at the same time, so that it becomes a habit.

Go somewhere quiet and warm, sit comfortably and close your eyes (you don't have to, but it will mean you are less likely to be distracted by things in the room).

The first thing to do is notice. How does your body feel? What emotions are you experiencing? What are you thinking about?

Thoughts will pop up. Let them come and go, but try not to get tangled up in them. Be an observer. Imagine you are sitting watching them play out like a movie.

Don't panic if strong emotions surface, as this is natural. Allow yourself to feel them fully so they can be released.

If you find yourself getting continually caught up in your thoughts, which most of us do, try the following simple techniques:

- Count your breaths. Go from 1 to 10 and repeat.

- Do a mental body scan. Begin with your feet and work your way slowly around the body, focusing on each part as you go.

- Listen to the sounds around you, whether it be birdsong, distant traffic or the wind against a window.

- Silently repeat a one-word mantra.

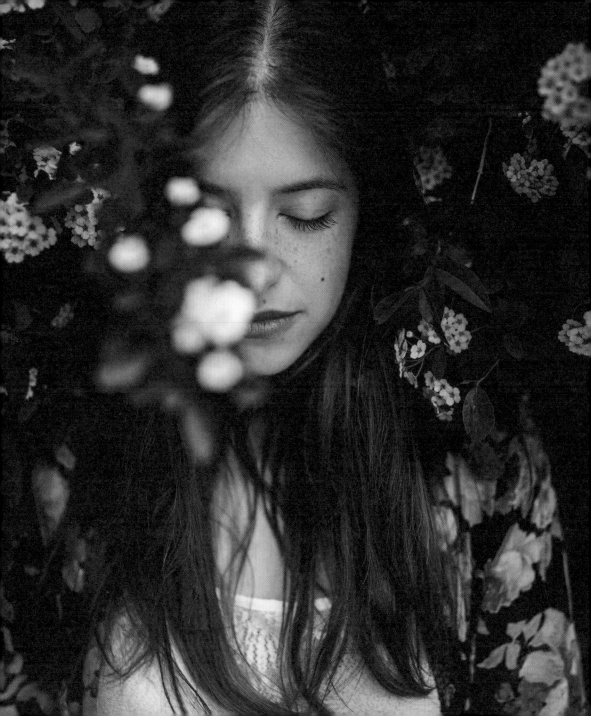

Mindfulness

Most of us veer between worrying about what lies ahead or ruminating on what happened in the past; it's a natural part of the human condition. Mindfulness is the practice of breaking free from this state and living in the present moment.

Mindfulness can reduce anxiety, release the grip of negative emotions and remind us of just how beautiful life on this planet can be. Every moment can be a mindful one, whether you are waiting for a bus, washing dishes or writing an email.

You don't have to make any big changes to your life or learn any complicated techniques, as everybody is born with the ability to be mindful. We do it naturally as children, but as we grow older, the burdens of adult life distract us.

Mindfulness is simply being aware of what is happening in the present moment – your thoughts, feelings and what is going on around you. You can start by trying some of the ideas on the next page – maybe even for just a few seconds, several times a day. Your mind will wander, but try not to get frustrated – it's been doing it for a lifetime and it will take time to encourage it to behave differently.

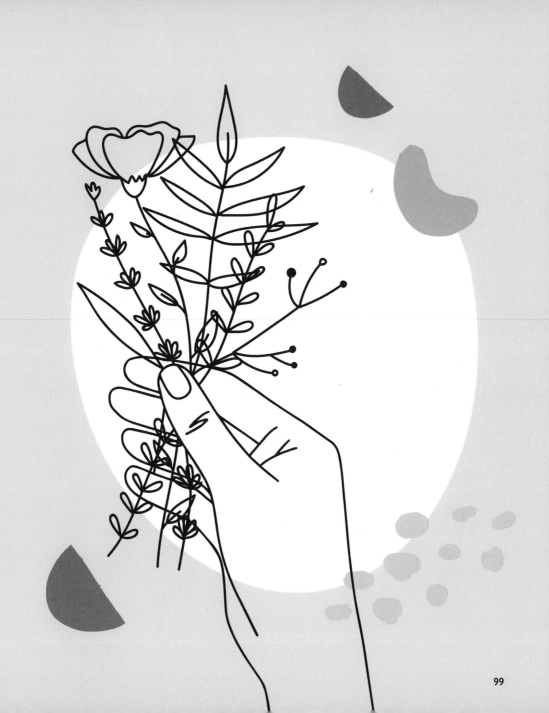

Daily mindfulness checklist

Things you can do each day in an effort to be more mindful:

- When you wake up in the morning, pay attention to your breathing and count five mindful breaths.

- If you find yourself in a queue, take a moment to feel the floor beneath your feet. Notice your feelings. Are you impatient? Angry?

- Bring awareness to tasks you normally do on autopilot. Slow down and notice everything that is happening, within and around you.

- If you have an overly busy mind, go for a walk in or near nature and look closely at your surroundings.

- Notice the times when you get sucked into worrying about the past or future.

- Bring awareness to your communication with others – can you be a better listener? Could you speak less? Pay attention to what you say.

- Wear a rubber band around your wrist as a reminder to be more mindful throughout the day. Every time you notice the band, think about your current state of mind. Are you fully immersed in the present or caught up in thinking about the past or future? If the latter is true, pull your focus back and sink into what is happening right now.

- Set an hourly alarm and each time it goes off, let yourself drop into present-moment awareness.

- Rather than gobble your food down, savour every mouthful. Notice the smell, texture and flavours of everything you consume.

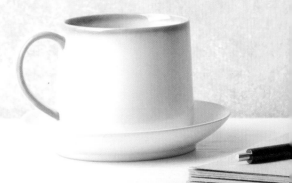

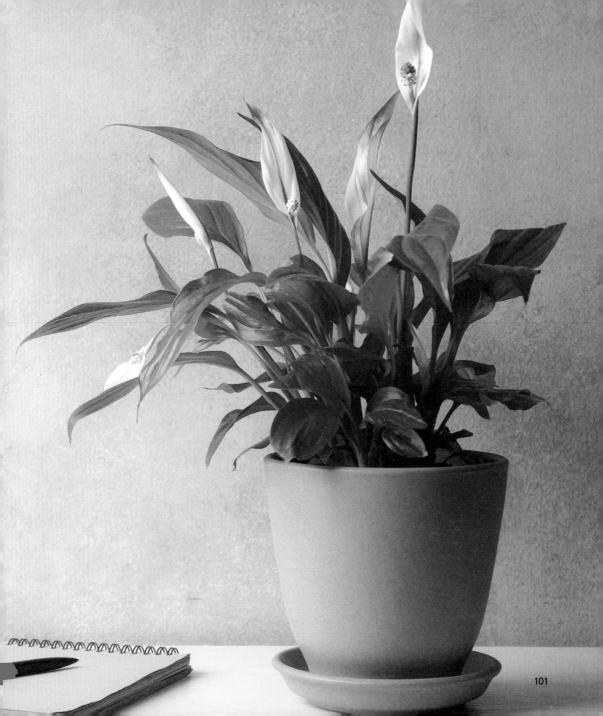

Grounding meditation

This simple grounding meditation is perfect for times when you are feeling overwhelmed by busyness or in a frenzied state of mind. It will bring you back down to earth in just a few minutes.

The exercise is devised to bring your awareness back to your body, your senses and the present moment.

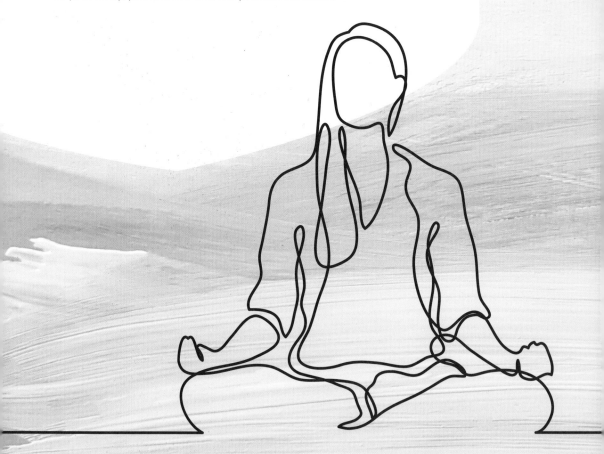

LEAVE YOUR MOBILE PHONE IN A DIFFERENT ROOM.

SIT COMFORTABLY SOMEWHERE YOU WON'T BE DISTURBED.

CLOSE YOUR EYES AND TAKE 10 DEEP BREATHS.
IMAGINE YOU ARE INHALING LIGHT AND HEALING ENERGY,
AND EXHALING HEAVINESS, STRESS AND WORRY.

CONCENTRATE ON YOUR FEET. CAN YOU FEEL THE
ENERGY COURSING THROUGH THEM? WHAT SENSATIONS
DO YOU NOTICE? DO THIS FOR 10 BREATHS.

NEXT, TURN YOUR ATTENTION TO YOUR HANDS
FOR 10 SLOW BREATHS. HOW DO THEY FEEL?
ARE THEY WARM? TINGLING? ACHEY?

REPEAT UNTIL YOU FEEL CALM AND PRESENT.

In this precise moment,
everything is OK and I
have no reason to worry

If we are not fully ourselves,
truly in the present moment,
we miss everything.

Thích Nhất Hạnh

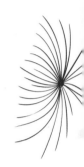
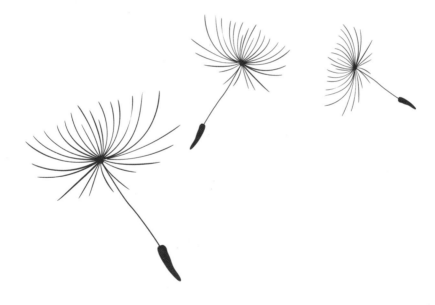

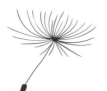

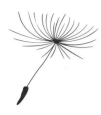

Breath work

We breathe 24/7 and rarely think about it, yet the amount of oxygen we take in affects every cell in our bodies. Many of us breathe badly without realizing: anxiety, poor posture and emotional blockages can make breathing shallow, which means we take in less oxygen and put the body under stress. Breath work aims to correct any abnormalities with our breathing patterns and has physical, mental and spiritual benefits.

Try this simple yogic breathing exercise:

- Sit comfortably in a chair and imagine that you are somewhere tranquil and relaxing.

- Inhale and exhale as deeply as you can 20 times.

- Let your breath return to normal.

- Sit with your eyes closed and notice how you feel – you should experience a greater sense of inner calm.

For maximum benefit, do this breathing technique for 10 minutes a day.

Whenever you feel anxious or stressed, pay attention to your breathing. If you notice that you are taking shallow breaths, make a conscious effort to slow down your breathing. This should result in a sensation of relaxation and calm.

Mantras

A mantra is a word or phrase that is repeated in a bid to clear the mind, improve mood and plant the seed of a positive intention. The things you think about can happen, so by focusing on an uplifting word or phrase, you are more likely to bring positive change into your life.

The first thing you need to do is choose a mantra that strikes a chord. You will know it's right as soon as you read or hear it.

Mantras were traditionally spoken in the ancient Sanskrit language. You could choose a traditional one, such as the word *om* (or *aum*) – the sacred sound of the universe that represents everything that is and ever was – or you can create your own. It might be as simple as "I am enough" or a single word such as "peace", "love" or "light".

Saying your mantra should become a habit. You can say it over and over while you meditate, write it on sticky notes and scatter them through the house, repeat it during yoga, in the bath – wherever you like! When you say the mantra repeatedly, it stills the thinking mind and makes it easier to access your higher self – that's the part of you that is most evolved and already knows the deepest truths.

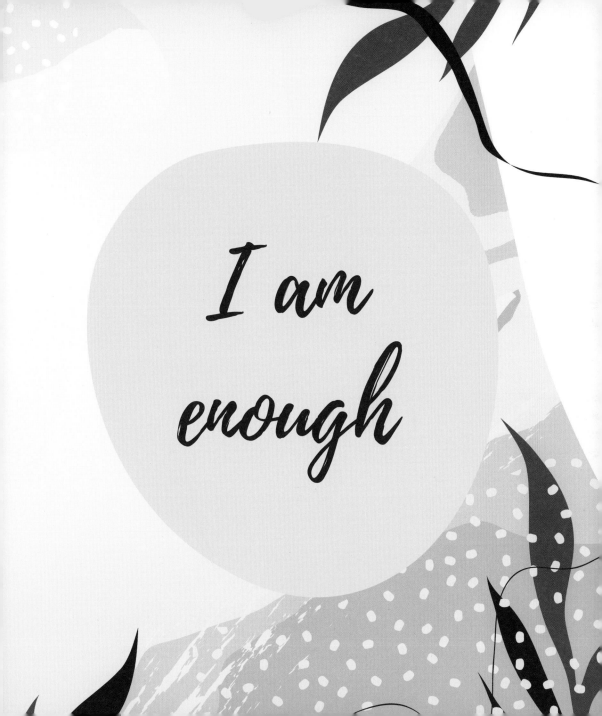

Affirmations

An affirmation is a positive statement that is designed to change the way you think by reprogramming the unconscious mind.

The words should relate to a specific goal you have in mind. For example, if you want to get fit you could say "I am getting stronger every day"; or if your finances need attention, you might choose the words "Money flows freely into my bank account".

Make sure the words are positive. For example, saying "I need more money" is focusing on lack and that won't inspire the positive emotions that are going to help you.

Repeat your affirmation as often as you can. You might feel silly at first, but if you keep saying it over and over with as much faith and passion as you can muster, you will start to believe it. This will result in changes in behaviour and attitude and you'll be a huge step closer to fulfilling your wishes.

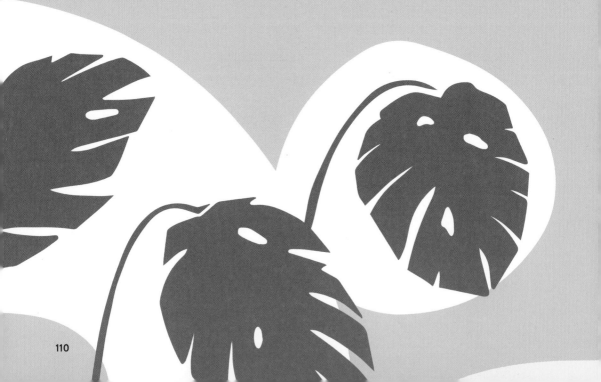

Here are a few examples of some positive affirmations:

Success and love come easily to me.

The universe has got my back.

My body is filled with healthy energy.

My health is getting better every day.

I deserve health and happiness.

Abundance flows to me.

Forgiveness

You might be wondering what forgiveness has got to do with well-being. Well the answer is a lot, as it happens. Forgiveness isn't about letting people trample all over you, it's about making a decision to let go of grudges and move on from events that happened in the past. Resentment is a powerful emotion and it's not good for you. When you hold a grudge, you tend to suffer a lot more than the person you are angry with.

Sometimes it can feel very difficult to forgive another, but once you make a conscious choice to do so, feelings of hurt and anger can be replaced by love, peace and happiness. There is an ancient Hawaiian practice that might help you forgive another called the Ho'oponopono Prayer. It operates on the basis that everything is connected and we are each responsible for what happens in our lives. If you are wronged, picture the other person and say: "I am sorry, forgive me. Thank you. I love you." The prayer will help you release resentment and foster forgiveness.

It's good for your health, too, as forgiveness has been linked with lower stress levels, better blood pressure, sleep quality and energy levels. Studies also show that people who practise the art of forgiveness, suffer from fewer illnesses.

If you are really struggling, write down all the reasons why you feel resentment toward a particular person or event. Don't hold back; let the words flow out. This can feel very cathartic. When you've finished, burn the paper, take a deep breath and vow to let it go, and then see if your heart is more open to forgiving the past.

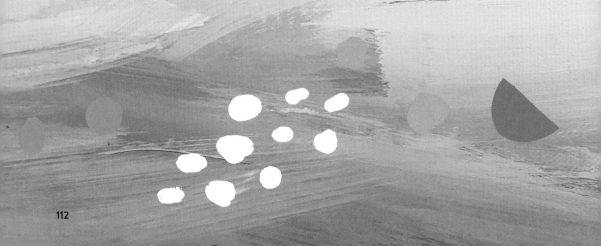

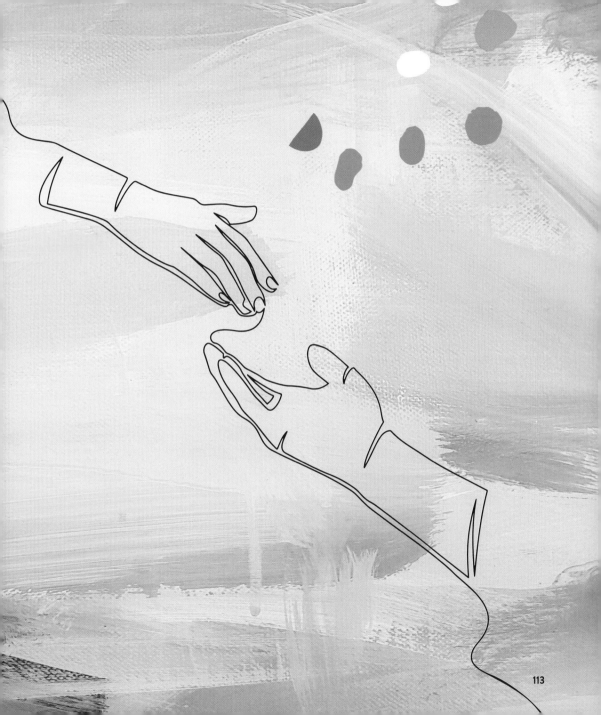

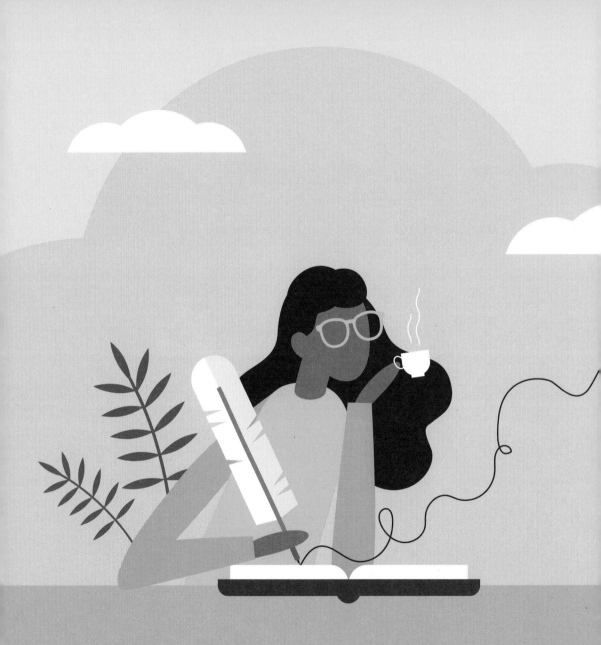

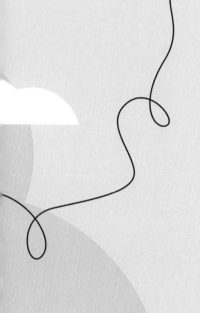

The gift of gratitude

Counting your blessings is such a simple thing to do and has enormous benefits for your mind, body and soul. When the going gets tough, it's easy to forget all the wonderful things we already have in our lives, but taking time out to appreciate them can fill you with warmth, happiness and a sense of abundance. It will leave you feeling more positive, which can only help you to attract more good things.

Make gratitude a habit and you'll soon start seeing the difference. Start a gratitude journal and each night, before you go to sleep, write down three things you were grateful for during the day. Make sure you name different things each time and you'll soon see how lucky you are.

Or you can choose an object as the focus of your gratitude. For example, you could use a pretty pebble that fits in the palm of your hand. Hold it for a few moments before you go to bed and think of three things you are thankful for.

Research has found that people who show a lot of gratitude are happier, have better relationships, are less likely to suffer from depression, and experience fewer aches and pains.

Transcendental meditation

Transcendental meditation was pioneered by Maharishi Mahesh Yogi, the notorious guru who instructed The Beatles. This style of meditation has been around for more than 50 years and can only be taught by certified teachers. You can find your nearest practitioner by visiting the official website at www.tm.org.

The practice involves sitting for 15–20 minutes twice a day and repeating a mantra silently in your head with your eyes closed. If thoughts take over, you gently bring your attention back to the mantra.

The term "transcendental" is used as the technique supposedly enables you to rise above the thinking mind and connect with your "higher self". During the session, the meditator will fall into a state that is between sleep and wakefulness.

There have been more than 650 scientific studies into the practice and it's proven that hospital visits are 50 per cent less frequent among those who practise transcendental meditation. Followers say that transcendental meditation reduces stress and gives them increased energy levels, clarity, and deeper levels of love and compassion. There are more than 10 million devotees across the globe, and the great thing is, it's relatively easy to master.

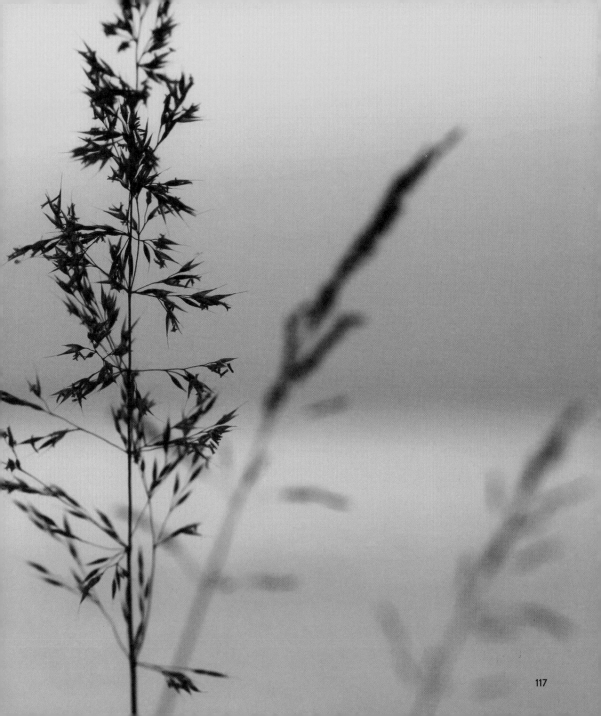

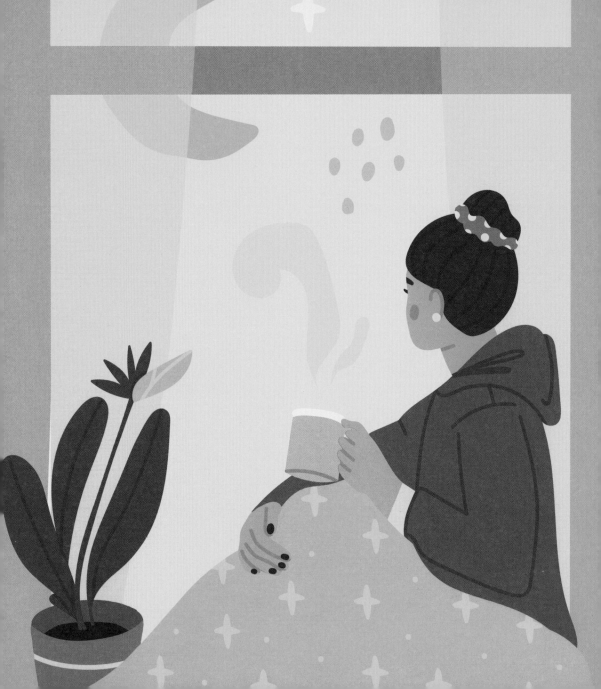

Silence is golden

Spiritual teachers say that spending time in silence is one of the most powerful ways of connecting with your soul. It also calms the mind, encourages the release of negative emotions and can really get your creative juices flowing.

It's about more than not talking. During therapeutic silence, you shouldn't be looking at your phone, reading books, watching TV or listening to music, as these things interrupt the process of quieting your busy mind. Picking up a magazine or sending a text will stimulate the brain too much. However, you can exercise, write, paint or draw – anything that is done peacefully and allows you to fall into a state of "flow", where your thoughts can start to slow down.

In our modern, noise-polluted, screen-obsessed culture where we are always switched on, silence has never been more necessary. While too much noise causes stress and tension, silence helps us to unwind and relax.

Still not convinced? How about this for a fact – a 2013 study showed that silence can encourage brain cells to regenerate!

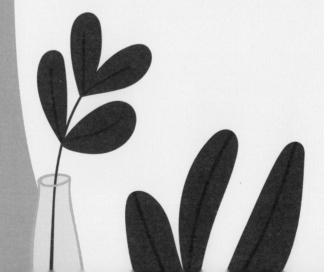

Silence on retreat or at home

You can practise silence at home or at an organized retreat with other people and an experienced facilitator.

At home you will need to switch off the phone, put a note on the front door to say please don't knock and make sure you are alone, as it is difficult to do this when you are surrounded by other people. If you live with others, ask them to give you some privacy for the next few hours.

Aim for a period of at least five hours in total silence. It is better if you can take a whole day off, as you may have to ease yourself gently back into the world of noise and constant stimulus afterwards.

There are no rules as to what you should be doing during the period of silence – anything goes as long it doesn't involve talking, looking at a screen or reading. If it helps, you can journal your thoughts and feelings, and it can be soothing to take a long, hot bath. Fresh air is essential, too, so try and take a quiet walk outdoors.

On a silent retreat, you will have a more structured experience of silence with the benefit of support from a facilitator. When you are alone with nothing but your own thoughts for company, long-buried emotions can be driven to the surface and it's helpful to have the guidance of a therapist at hand. There is also something freeing about being with others and not having to think of things to say!

When looking for a silent retreat, choose somewhere in a location you will find restful. Many centres ask that you share a room and pitch in with chores, which might be an easier transition for those who usually like to stay busy, but there are some retreats that offer single occupancy and no requirements for you to do any work – pick one that suits you.

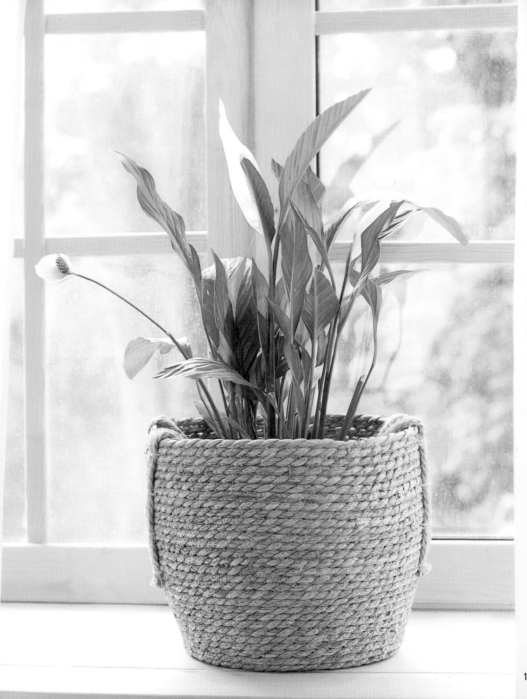

The power of thought

You are what you think you are, so if you want your life to be different, you have to change your mind. Naturally, positive thoughts are much more conducive to a happy life than negative ones.

We all know those glass-half-empty people who moan about life at any given opportunity and from the outside they may seem to have it bad. Likewise, there's the glass-half-full brigade who see the positive in any given situation and appear to be born lucky.

Our minds are like magnets – we attract what we put out – but it is difficult to stay positive when life gets taxing. It's worth making the effort though, as science shows that our brains rewire themselves to turn repetitive thoughts into habits, so the more upbeat thinking you do the better. Happiness is a choice.

Here are a few things that can help you stay positive:

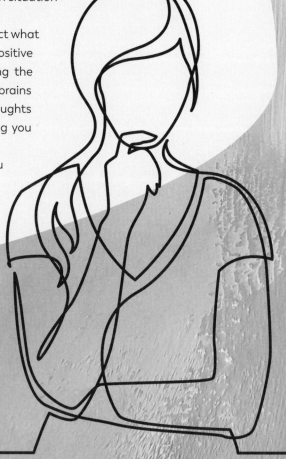

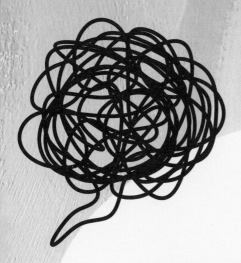

- **Meditate regularly** – take just 10 minutes each day to sit quietly and do nothing.

- **Be thankful** – jot down the things that you are grateful for.

- **Be kind** – when you are about to react to another person, stop for a moment and consider what the kindest course of action would be.

- **Get plenty of me time** – do things you love!

- **Try not to worry too much** – this is easier said than done, but worries only persist if we fuel them with thoughts. Try to spend as much time as you can in the present moment, where unless you face immediate danger there is never much to worry about.

- **Be your own biggest fan!** – be kind to yourself and instead of concentrating on your failures, celebrate every victory no matter how small.

Chapter Six

Home-Grown Holistic Therapy

The beauty of holistic therapy is that it urges each of us to take responsibility for our own health, and there are a range of things we can do for ourselves at home at very little expense. Unlike conventional medicine, which requires years of training before you can practise, holistic healing is gentle and safe, and there is no reason why you cannot treat yourself – although, you should always seek the advice of your doctor first if you have any concerning health issues.

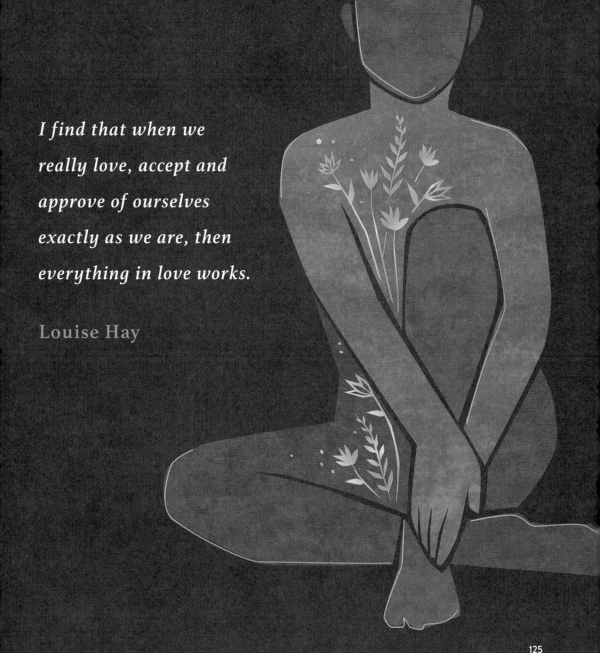

I find that when we really love, accept and approve of ourselves exactly as we are, then everything in love works.

Louise Hay

Nature is the best medicine

Studies have shown that being in and around nature really does heal us – even looking at pictures of the natural world can reduce stress and anxiety and lower blood pressure. Some hospitals use vast murals of outdoor scenes in their wards and waiting rooms for this very reason. With our busy lifestyles that involve spending a lot of time staring at screens, it's more important than ever to make sure we get outdoors if we can.

There is nothing quite like the sun on your skin, the wind in your hair, the sound of birdsong, and the sight of flora and fauna to lift the spirits. You don't have to live in the wilderness to get your dose of nature. A walk around your local park, nearby beauty spots or even sitting in the garden and admiring the view will be hugely beneficial.

When you are out in nature, try to appreciate it fully. Look closely at the trees and the plants, and look out for wildlife. Take time to smell any pretty blooms, touch leaves and bark, listen to the sound of plants rustling in the wind, and if the mood takes you, why not hug a tree? Many people find it to be really grounding.

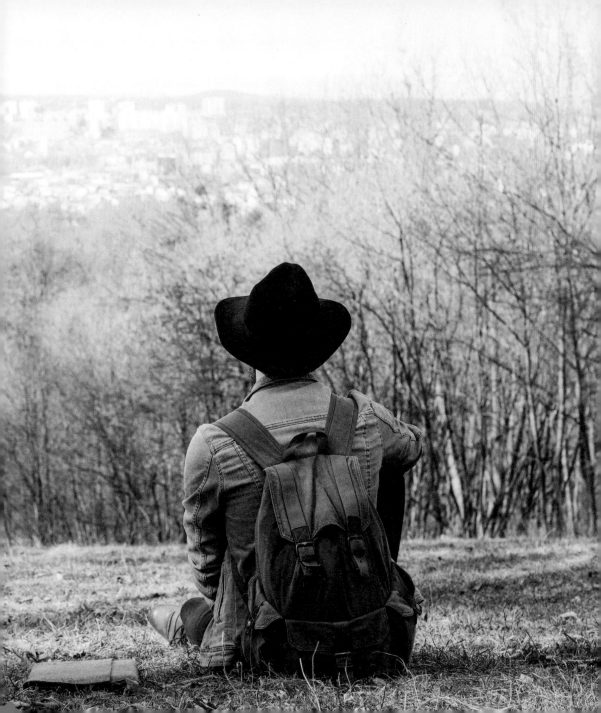

Grow things

There's nothing like growing plants, flowers or vegetables from seed to make you appreciate the miracle of life on this planet. Hold a single seed in the palm of your hand and it appears to be an unremarkable thing, but give it soil, water and sunlight, and watch as life shoots forth before your very eyes.

Research shows that getting your hands dirty in soil is great for your mood as it can increase serotonin levels – that's a feel-good hormone produced by the body. It's a natural antidepressant and it strengthens the immune system.

If you don't have outdoor space, you can always put some pots on your windowsill. Herbs such as basil, oregano and parsley will thrive when grown indoors, as long as they are in pots with good drainage and have at least six hours of sunlight per day; and vegetables such as chard, potatoes and cucumber will also grow well when potted.

When it comes to harvesting your crops, researchers have found that picking food you have grown or foraged yourself can produce a dopamine hit. That's another happy hormone that is released in the brain causing a feeling of bliss. That's before you've even tasted the fruits of your labour!

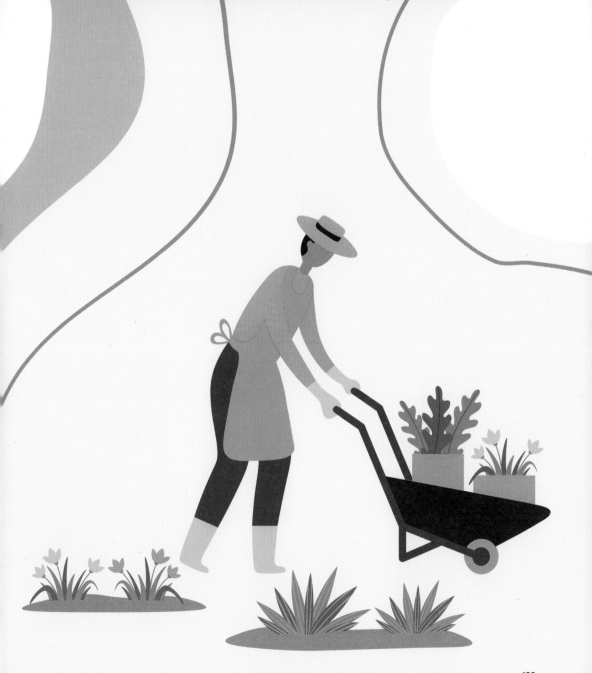

Drinking water

I know, you've heard it all before: drink, drink, drink. But do you really need to keep knocking back water all day? The answer is a big fat YES. Water is essential for your health; it makes up two-thirds of your bodyweight and without it you wouldn't survive the week. Research suggests that if the level of fluids in your body drops by just 1 per cent it may reduce brainpower. Drinking too little will also affect energy levels and emotions.

Everybody is different and the best way to find out if you are drinking enough is to look at your pee. It should be very light yellow or clear in colour. If it is dark, you may be dehydrated.

Experts say that it is best to drink little and often, and most of us should aim for between six to eight glasses of water and other liquids each day. Tea, coffee and soft drinks count, but nothing is better for you than water. If you find pure old-fashioned water dull, try adding a sprig of mint, some crushed ice, lime, lemon or orange to it. Experiment and find something that works for you.

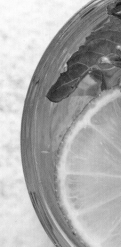

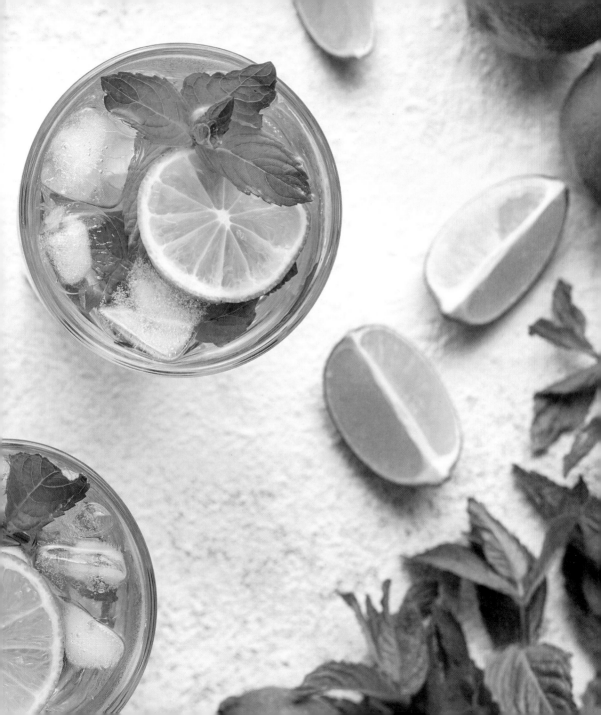

Life is a wonderful adventure and I am open to trying new and enriching things

In today's rush we all think
too much, seek too much, want
too much and forget about
the joy of just being.

Eckhart Tolle

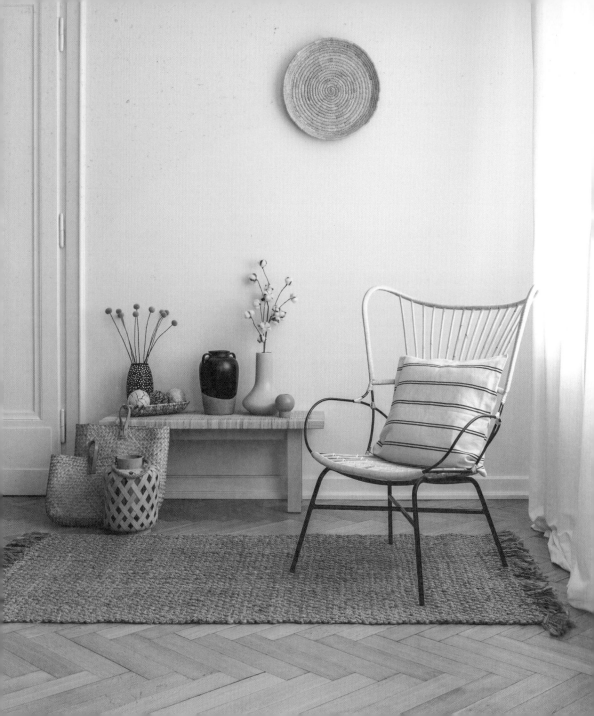

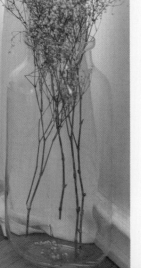

An allergen-free home

No matter how clean you keep your home, there are tiny particles in the air such as dust, mould or pollen that can trigger hayfever, asthma symptoms or other allergic reactions. Here are a few ways you can remove allergens for a happier, healthier home:

- Dust mites are one of the biggest offenders when it comes to allergies in the home, and to combat them you should cover your pillow and mattress with dust mite covers.

- If you react strongly to dust, consider replacing carpets with wooden floors and if you do have carpets, make sure that your vacuum cleaner has a HEPA (high-efficiency particulate air) filter that can trap minute particles.

- Make sure you wash curtains regularly (around every 6 months) and if you have blinds, vacuum and wipe them regularly with a wet cloth.

- To banish mould, ventilate the bathroom, clean it regularly and replace silicon and caulk at least every few years. Kill any visible mould with diluted bleach.

- Always clear mould from the fridge, clean out your food waste caddies regularly and check your walls, plumbing and windows for any signs of damp or leaks.

Friendships

Experts say that we are experiencing a loneliness epidemic, which is ironic considering that smartphones and tablets mean we are always connected to each other. But the 400 friends you might have on Facebook or Instagram pale into insignificance when compared with a true bestie; someone who loves you warts and all, who makes you laugh and will pick you up if you fall. The benefits of friendship are well documented: a study by Harvard University concluded that having good friends makes us healthier, mentally and physically.

It's just one of many reasons to nurture your current friendships and be open to the possibility of making new ones. There's no need to worry about accumulating dozens of pals because British anthropologist Robin Dunbar says that while the average person can maintain 150 social friendships, we are only able to maintain three to five close friends at any one time.

If you need an excuse to cherish your inner circle, here are five reasons why friends are good for you:

- Friends have helped to shape the person you are today.

- You learn great life skills from your close friends.

- Having friends makes life easier – not only in the emotional support they provide, but they can also help you meet a partner, advance your career or inspire you.

- When we form friendships with people who are different from us, we have an opportunity to stretch ourselves and learn new things.

- The friendship you give to others benefits them enormously – it's one of the greatest gifts you can give a person.

So, what are you waiting for? Call your best friend now and tell them how great they are!

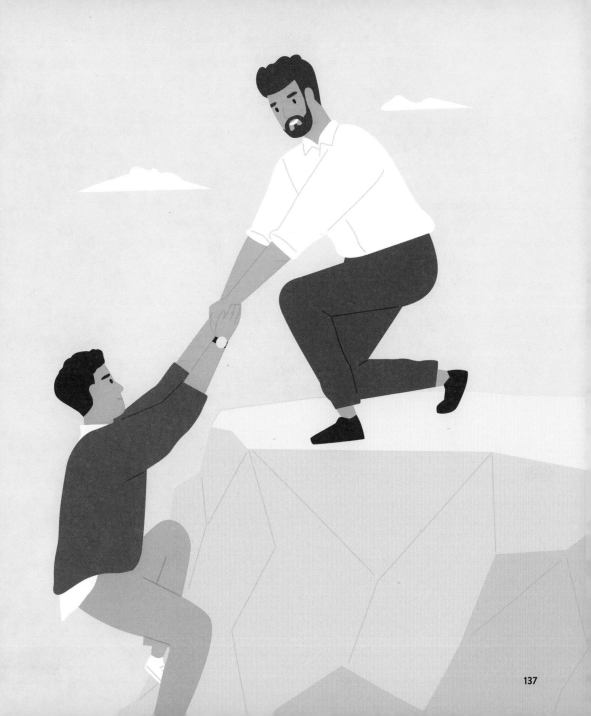

Self-love

Have you heard the saying "If you don't love yourself, you can't love another"? Well, it's true. What you feel inside, you give out, and if you only follow one piece of advice in this book, make it falling in love with yourself.

You are the only you on this planet. That makes you truly special. You're amazing and you need to know that.

We've all got an inner critic that tells us we are not good enough, have messed up again or will never achieve our dreams. That voice is lying. Don't listen to it. The more you ignore it, the quieter it gets.

Here are a few simple ways you can be your own best friend and cultivate self-love:

- Begin each day by making a positive statement about yourself.

- Think about someone you really admire. What quality of theirs do you love? Remind yourself that you are only attracted to this person because they reflect what is already in you!

- Stop comparing yourself with others.

- List all your good qualities and the things that make you unique.

- Learn to say "no" and set clear boundaries. Putting yourself first is not selfish.

- If you mess up, forgive yourself as you would a small child. We all make mistakes!

- Be aware of the voice inside your head – would you talk to a friend like that?

- Know that all the love you will ever need is inside you right now.

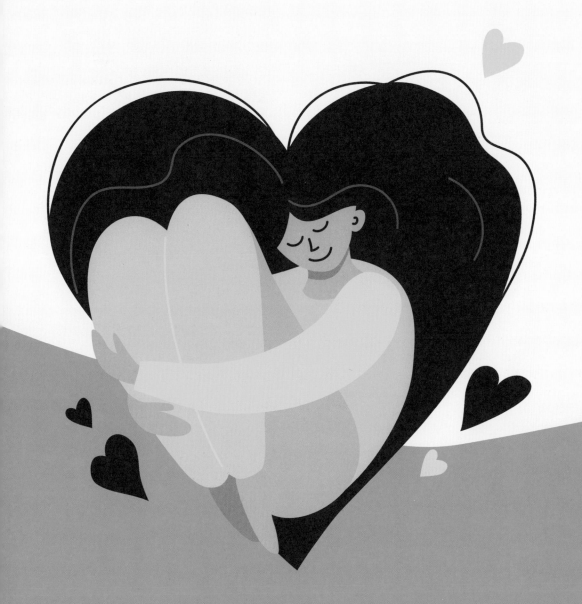

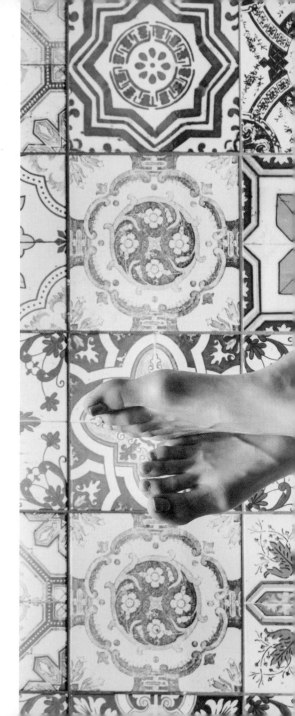

Create a
sacred space

It is important that we spend a little time alone with ourselves in silence every day. A good way to turn this into a habit that you want to keep is to create a sacred space in your home. This will be a sanctuary that you can retreat to when you need to find a bit of inner stillness. For that reason, it should make you feel calm, uplifted and happy – a messy junk room or a spot next to the washing machine isn't going to cut it! If you share your home, make sure you pick a spot where you can have some privacy and let others know the importance of your sacred space.

Some people like to place religious icons in their sacred space – a statue of Buddha or a Hindu god, perhaps – while others opt for a candle, crystals or some pretty flowers and coloured silks. We're all different and only you know how to create a sacred space that works for you.

To make it extra soothing, try putting a few drops of essential oil in a plant mister with some water and give your space a spritz before you settle down.

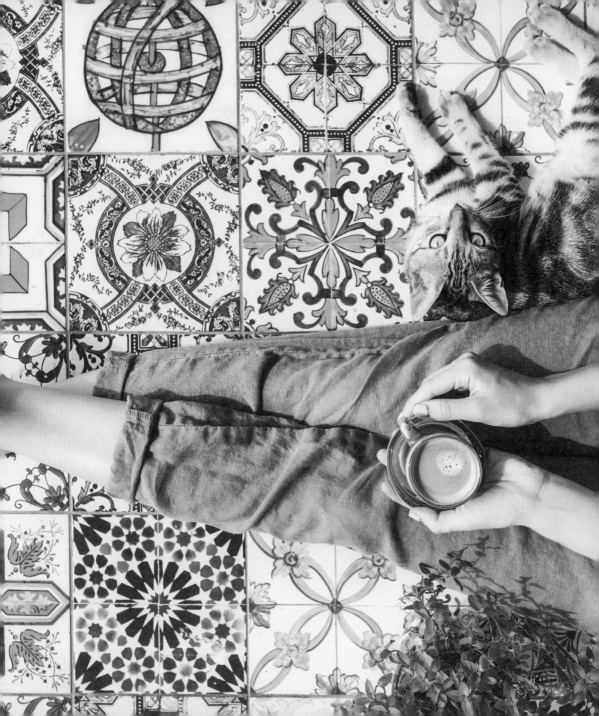

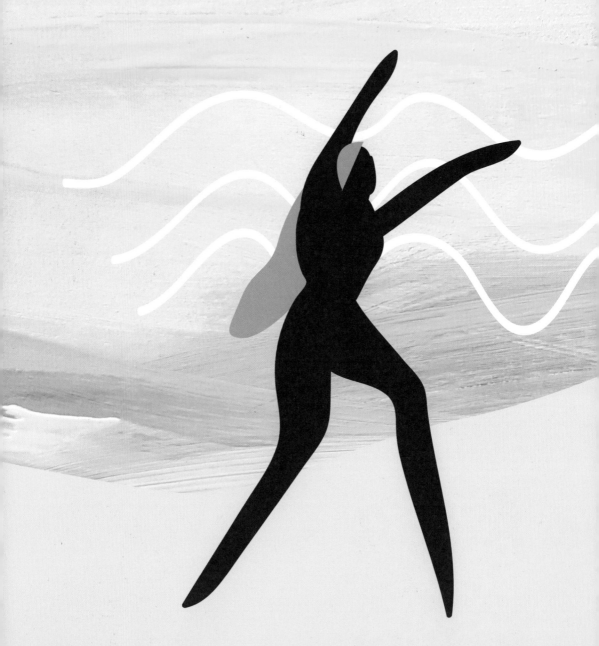

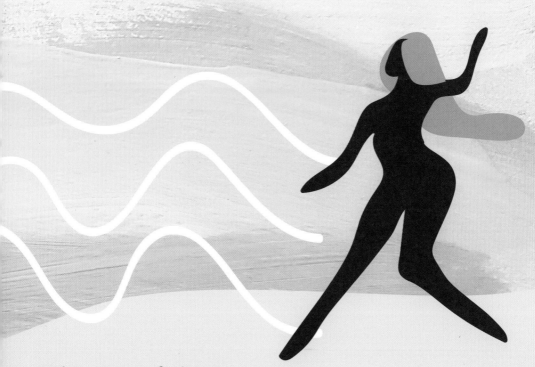

The joy of dance

Research shows that in addition to improving fitness levels, dancing is good for mental health, too – it improves mood and relieves stress and anxiety. You don't have to be a fantastic mover to reap the benefits of dance. Letting yourself go and moving to a favourite piece of music can be a fast-track to happiness.

There are so many forms of dance to choose from. You can rock out to heavy metal in your bedroom or find a class in anything you fancy, from ballet through to flamenco, hip hop or tap. If you feel shy about performing in front of others or there aren't any classes near you, you can always try one of the many free online dance classes that are available – it's even possible to take part in silent discos on the internet with others across the globe.

Remember, unless you actually earn your living as a dancer, it doesn't matter what you look like while you're dancing; it's about how moving to music makes you feel.

Walking to happiness

If you are able to walk, then you have an instant form of therapy always to hand: the benefits and rewards of walking are many. There's no need for long hikes either, unless that's your thing, because you only need to walk for 30 minutes a day to improve your health.

Here's what you'll gain from making walking a regular part of your day:

- Walking will keep your heart healthy and reduce the risk of having a stroke by up to 27 per cent.

- It releases feel-good hormones, which lift the mood and can help fend off depression.

- It strengthens the bones.

- Regular exercise such as walking has been shown to add up to eight years on to your life expectancy.

- A brisk half-hour walk can burn up to 200 calories – that adds up to 0.5 kg (1 lb) in bodyweight in 17 days.

- For women, it reduces the risk of breast cancer by 14 per cent.

- Getting outdoors will ensure you get a regular boost of vitamin D – the average person needs 10–20 minutes of midday sunlight several times a week to keep the levels topped up (just make sure you don't let your skin start to redden!).

- Regular exercisers are around 50 per cent less likely to catch a cold.

- Walking improves your balance.

- It is thought that the risk of Alzheimer's is halved if you get regular physical exercise. Walking just 5 miles a week has been shown to help prevent the disease and physical activity can also slow deterioration in those already experiencing cognitive decline.

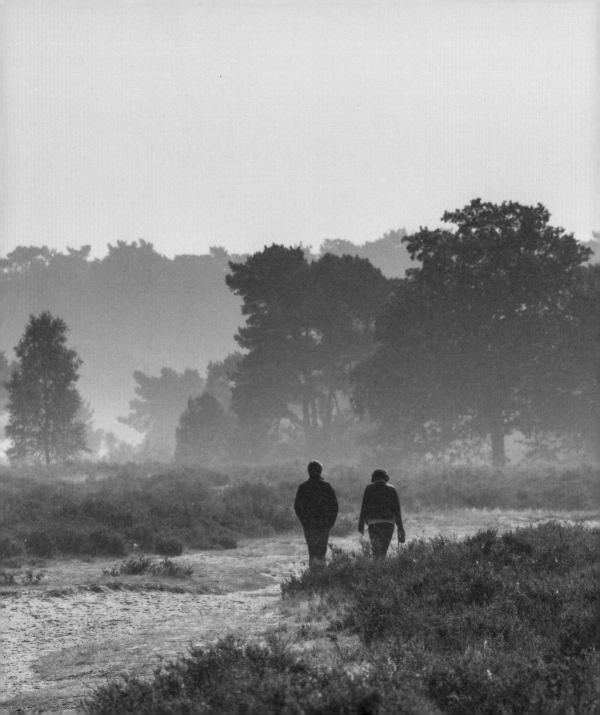

Barefoot benefits

There are obvious practical benefits to wearing shoes, but taking them off and going barefoot has lots of advantages as long as you are careful where you step.

Feeling grass, earth or sand beneath your feet is both uplifting and grounding, but it's also good for your posture and for your feet. There are more nerves in the feet than any other part of the body, which means that when you exercise barefoot, more information is fed back to the brain and this really helps with balance.

Barefoot walking and running strengthens the feet and the calf muscles, and can help improve conditions such as flat feet and bunions. It can also lead to a wider range of hip movements. Plus, when you walk or run barefoot, you have to concentrate on each step, which means you are naturally being more mindful. So next time you're in a garden or park or on the beach, take off those shoes and embrace the power of your bare feet!

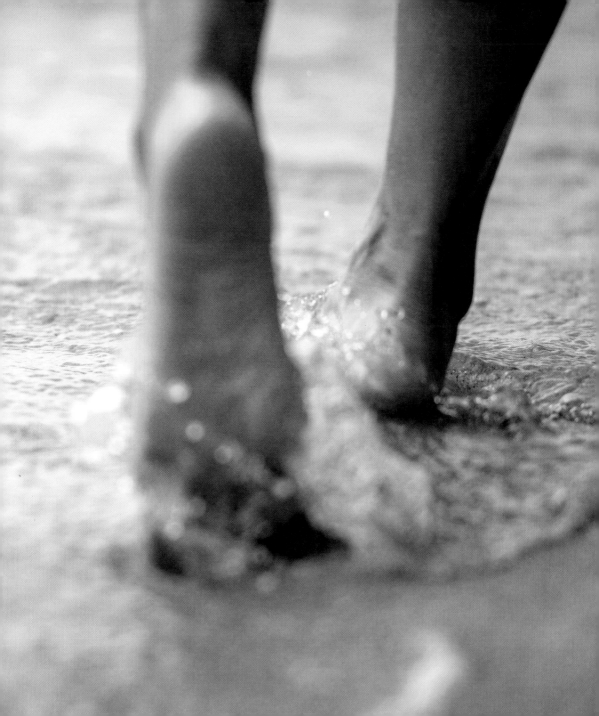

Vision boards

Visualization is one of the most powerful mental exercises you can do and research shows that it really works. Computer specialist Natan Sharansky spent hours in solitary confinement imagining himself becoming a world chess champion and that's exactly what happened when he beat Garry Kasparov in 1996.

Everything we create in our lives begins as a thought, and when you visualize something, you amplify that thought and train the mind to achieve it. Studies show that thinking about something creates similar brain patterns to those that occur if you actually do it – for example, you can actually work out your muscles by imagining yourself at the gym! With this in mind, it makes sense to create a vision board of all the things you would like to achieve in life. Just by looking at it, you are developing the mental strength to make it happen. Your vision board shouldn't just be a display of the things you want, it should sum up how you'd like to feel, too. What you put on that board is what you'll attract into your life.

To create your vision board:

1. Get a large piece of card.

2. Find pictures or words that represent the things you want in life.

3. Stick the images and words on to the board.

4. Hang the board in a place where you will see it and be inspired daily.

Your vision board will serve as a reminder of how you want your best life to be and looking at it regularly will help to reprogramme your subconscious so that you are primed to react to the right opportunities. Get tied up with too many negative thoughts and you might not even notice such opportunities, even when they are right in front of you.

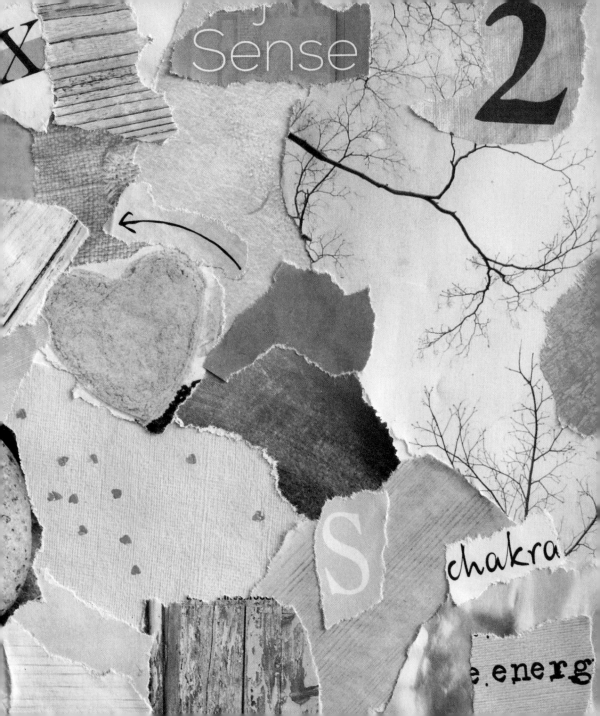

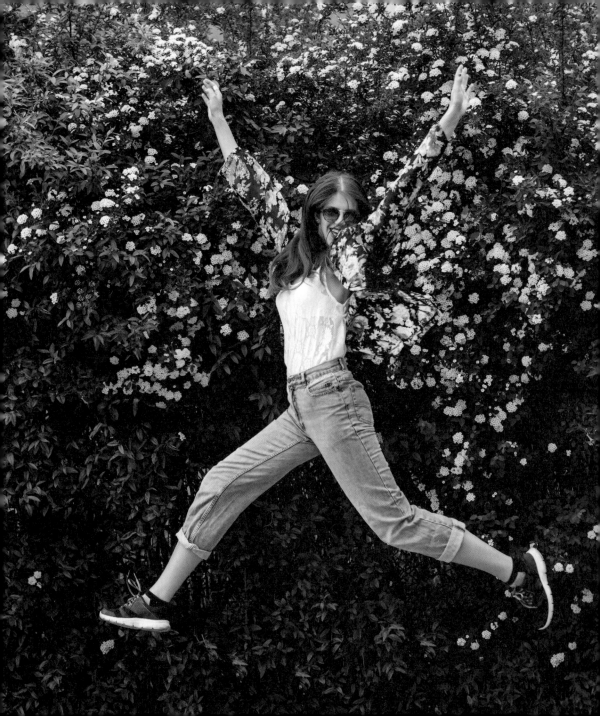

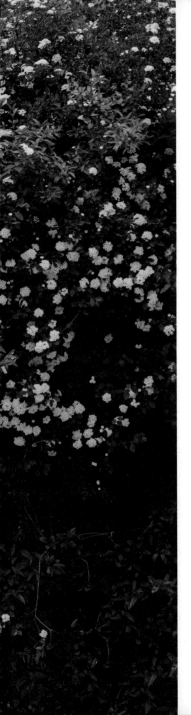

Try something new

We all get set in our ways, but a great way to change perspective, unleash creativity and generate new ideas is to do something completely new. This doesn't mean you have to take up abseiling or learn about quantum physics (unless that's your bag), as it can be as simple as taking a different route to the bus stop or trying a food you've never eaten before.

Life is so much more of an adventure when you keep trying out new stuff, and the chances are you'll discover passions and interests that have up until now remained hidden. See what new perspectives and ideas await you when you try something new.

- **Confidence** – trying something new will give you a real confidence boost.

- **New skills** – there is always so much to learn from all new endeavours.

- **Beat boredom** – doing new stuff can help lift you out of a rut.

- **Self-discovery** – you'll learn new things about yourself.

- **Friendships** – experimenting will mean you can meet people from different circles and make new friends.

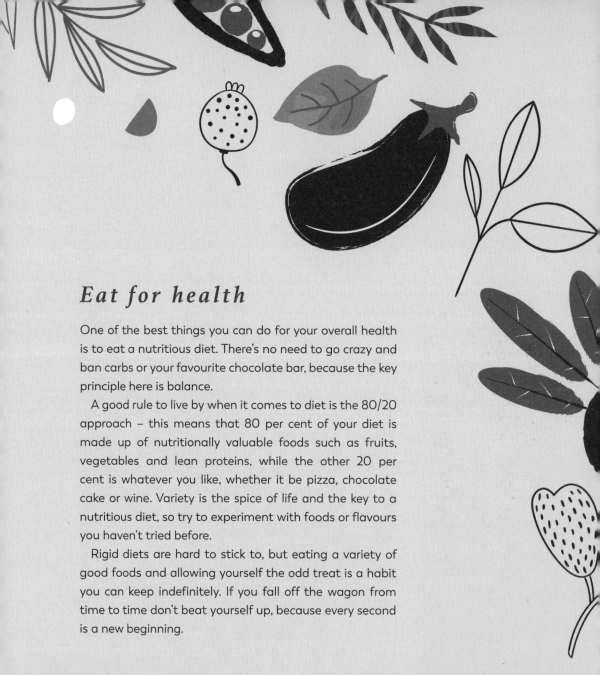

Eat for health

One of the best things you can do for your overall health is to eat a nutritious diet. There's no need to go crazy and ban carbs or your favourite chocolate bar, because the key principle here is balance.

A good rule to live by when it comes to diet is the 80/20 approach – this means that 80 per cent of your diet is made up of nutritionally valuable foods such as fruits, vegetables and lean proteins, while the other 20 per cent is whatever you like, whether it be pizza, chocolate cake or wine. Variety is the spice of life and the key to a nutritious diet, so try to experiment with foods or flavours you haven't tried before.

Rigid diets are hard to stick to, but eating a variety of good foods and allowing yourself the odd treat is a habit you can keep indefinitely. If you fall off the wagon from time to time don't beat yourself up, because every second is a new beginning.

I love my body and choose
to fill it with nutritious
foods, take exercise
and get ample rest

Food has the power to heal us. It is the most potent tool we have to help prevent and treat many of our chronic diseases.

Dr Mark Hyman

Conclusion

We can never control everything that happens to us in life, but we can take responsibility for our own health and well-being.

You are a child of nature living in an incredible body, which is mind-boggling in its complexity. You don't need to understand how it all works; all you need to do is ensure that your mind, body and spirit are in harmony.

This means paying attention to what your body is telling you and never neglecting any aspect of your life – where you live, your work, your relationships, what you read, the food you eat, the thoughts you have... they all add to the overall picture of your health.

There are so many holistic practices out there that can make us all feel better, with tons of elements that you can try for yourself at home; but if you only do one thing for yourself, become your own biggest fan. If you love and honour yourself and take time out to rest and listen to your body, you'll be the best and most brilliant version of yourself – and it would be unfair to deny the world that, wouldn't it?

And, finally, if you do have a bad day where you've eaten unhealthy foods, haven't moved from the sofa or have spent hours stressing about work, don't panic. Nobody is perfect and being your best self takes effort, otherwise everybody would be doing it. You're only human, be kind to yourself and know that you're doing a great job. Go you!

I am the creator of my
own health and choose
to be happy, whole
and fit every day

IMAGE CREDITS

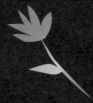

If you're interested in finding out more about our books,
find us on Facebook at **Summersdale Publishers**
and follow us on Twitter at **@Summersdale**.

www.summersdale.com